total
pilates

total
pilates

malcolm muirhead

editorial consultant yvonne worth

MQP

Published by MQ Publications Limited

12 The Ivories, 6-8 Northampton Street

London N1 2HY

Tel: 020 7359 2244

Fax: 020 7359 1616

email: mail@mqpublications.com

SERIES EDITORS: Kate John, Karen Ball MQ Publications

EDITORIAL DIRECTOR: Ljiljana Baird, MQ Publications

PHOTOGRAPHY BY Mike Prior

DESIGN BY Balley Design Associates

ILLUSTRATION BY gerardgraphics.co.uk

ISBN 1-84072-437-4

Printed in China

1 3 5 7 9 0 8 6 4 2

introduction to pilates

The Pilates method, which was first devised in the mid-1920s, was one of the first exercise systems in the West to take a holistic approach to fitness and well-being. The current trend for health and fitness and an ever-growing awareness of the importance of looking after ourselves on all levels—body, mind, and spirit—may explain the growing popularity of Pilates over recent years.

The Pilates technique offers a unique method of body control and conditioning—stretching and strengthening the muscles, while improving flexibility and balance. It does not require you to give up your current fitness routine. On the contrary, Pilates is an invaluable system that works in conjunction with other exercise programs, strengthening, realigning, and rebalancing the body, improving body awareness, and reducing risk of injury or strain.

To fully benefit from the Pilates system, it is essential to not only master the movements and to commit to a regular practice routine, but also to examine your current lifestyle and be

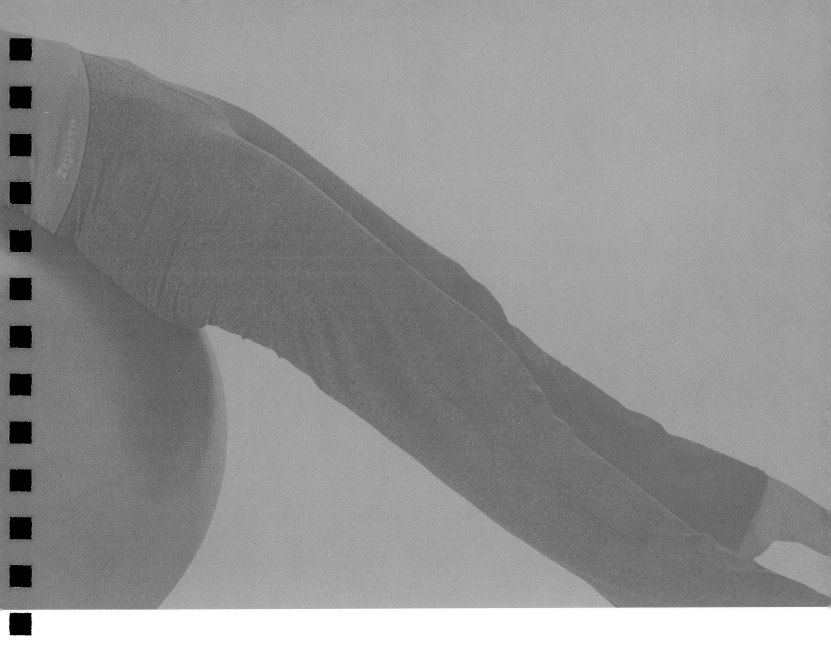

prepared to make changes where necessary. On a practical level, this involves making sure you get enough rest and eat a healthy diet, as well as maintaining your level of fitness and well-being, reducing stress, and keeping a positive outlook on life.

The Pilates technique helps you learn to recognize your strengths and your weaknesses and work toward rebalancing your body. The moves themselves function differently from many other forms of exercise. Here the focus is primarily on strengthening the central core and using the abdominal muscles to control the movements, whereas many other forms of strengthening exercise concentrate purely on developing the limbs themselves. Pilates works to stretch and lengthen the muscles, allowing the body to become stronger and firmer, without building bulk. It teaches you to focus the mind as you exercise the body, gradually improving your coordination, body awareness, flexibility, and overall alignment.

why pilates?

Pilates has been in existence since the 1920s and has always been favored by actors, dancers, performers, and athletes, but it is only in recent years that it has gained celebrity status and soared in popularity. As a result, many health and fitness centers now offer classes and some even have their own Pilates studios.

Some people are drawn to Pilates because of its proven body-shaping effects—the gentle stretching and lengthening movements draw the muscles into longer, leaner shapes. Others are drawn to it because they want a challenging whole-body workout that strengthens and increases stamina, but do not wish to lift weights. Still others are referred to Pilates by their chiropractor, osteopath, physical therapist, or medical practitioner.

Many people who have sustained a back or neck injury are drawn to Pilates, discovering it to be an excellent method of strengthening the body and preventing it from sustaining further injury.

The Pilates method is intended to complement any other fitness program you may be involved in, not replace it. Unlike other, more dynamic formats, such as dancing, aerobics, spinning, or other cardiovascular exercises, Pilates is not a system that necessarily causes the body temperature to rise or the circulation to increase. Therefore, when embarking on a Pilates program, it is recommended that you also take up some kind of cardiovascular exercise, if you have not already done so. This does not need to take the form of hefty aerobics classes; swimming or brisk walking would be equally effective.

Pilates is a subtle technique that works at supporting and protecting the body as you exercise. However, if you have any specific complaint, suffer chronic pain or discomfort, or have sustained any injuries, particularly to the spine or neck, then you should seek medical advice before embarking on any exercise program.

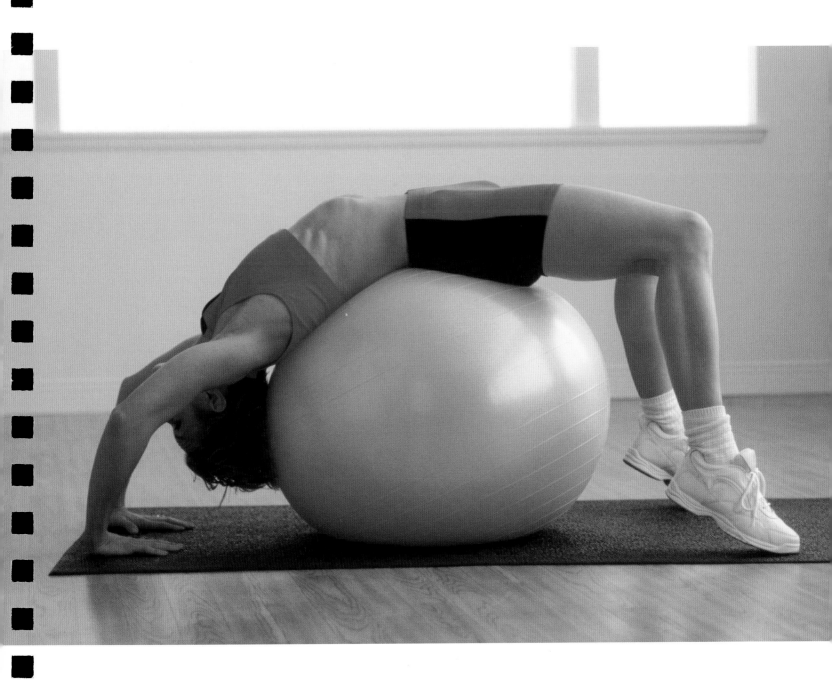

above: The exercise ball helps Pilates practitioners stretch their bodies without putting undue strain on joints and muscles.

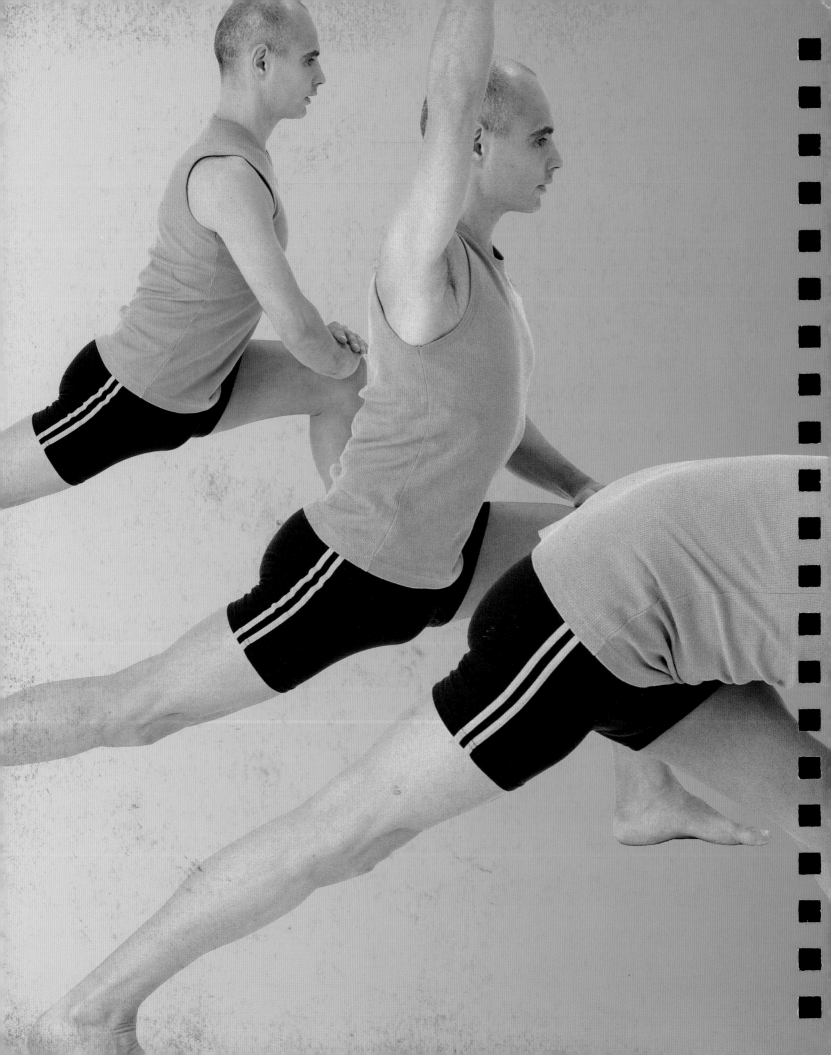

principles of pilates

benefits of pilates

Safety while exercising is an important aspect of any fitness regimen. However, many injuries occur in everyday life, for example, pulling muscles while lifting shopping bags or small children. The Pilates system retrains the body, increasing strength and flexibility and improving balance, posture, alignment, and muscle control. Consequently we become better able to manage our daily activities efficiently and effectively with little or no risk of strain or injury. Under the Pilates system, the body is worked as a whole, ensuring that stability, balance, correct alignment, good muscle control, and correct breathing are maintained while the various muscle groups are being exercised.

The Pilates system increases our self-awareness, making us more aware of what we unconsciously do with our bodies and enabling us to identify and alter bad habits. It also provides us with the opportunity to develop areas that need attention, allowing us to build up strength in our weak areas.

The key benefits of the Pilates method are as follows:
• Develops core abdominal strength
• Helps you develop a leaner body by lengthening and stretching the muscles without building bulk
• Improves balance, poise, stability, and flexibility
• Reduces stress and fatigue
• Works with the deepest muscles of the body to build strength and control
• Improves mind/body awareness
• Exercises the muscles without causing pain or risking muscle tear or jarred joints
• Teaches you not to strain your muscles, but to enjoy the movements as you stretch
• Enhances muscle control without causing tension
• Relieves pain, stiffness, and tension
• It is suitable for anyone, regardless of age or level of fitness
• The principles of Pilates can be applied to any movement or activity

The Pilates technique does not require you to buy any special equipment, although some basic equipment is available should you choose to purchase it. All you need is a folded blanket, towel, or exercise mat to place on the floor; a small towel, scarf, or stretchy exercise band; and a small, flat cushion to place under your head, if needed. Clothing should be comfortable and allow you to move freely.

caution: If you are pregnant or suffer from any illness or injury, you should seek medical advice before beginning any exercise program.

below: Pilates fits easily into your everyday life and can be practiced at home or in a class.

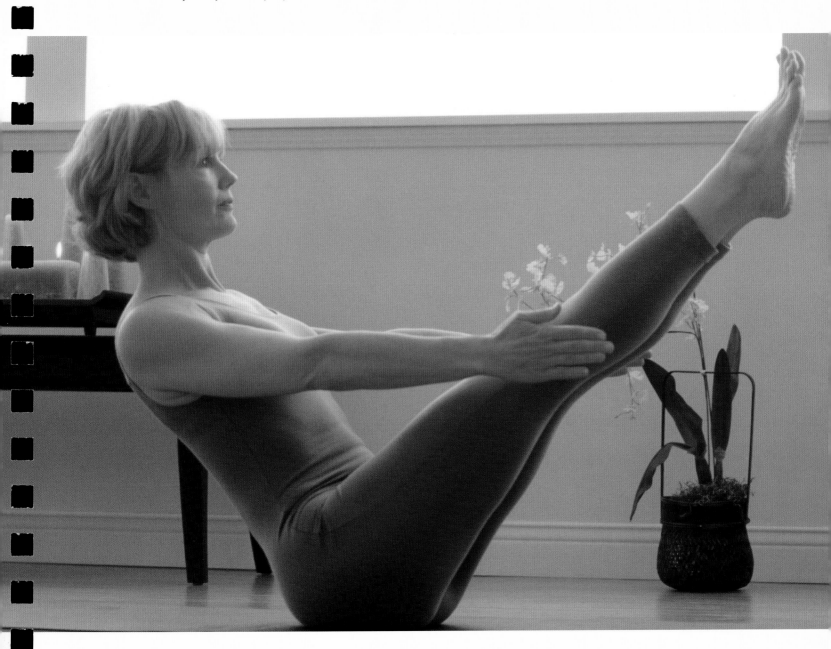

history

Joseph Pilates was born near Dusseldorf, Germany, in 1880. He was a sickly child, suffering from a variety of ailments, including asthma, rickets, and rheumatic fever. Determined to overcome his physical weakness, he dedicated himself to becoming physically fit and strong. He studied and became proficient at various activities, including bodybuilding, diving, skiing, and gymnastics. By the time he was fourteen years old he had become so physically fit that he was able to work as a model for anatomical charts.

In 1912, Pilates moved to the U.K., where he worked as a boxer, circus performer, and a self-defense trainer to detectives. During World War I, he was taken prisoner of war because of his nationality. Initially placed in a camp in Lancaster, as the war progressed, Pilates was moved to another camp on the Isle of Man. Here he became a hospital nurse and developed a fitness routine for the other internees. He began constructing equipment, removing bed springs and attaching them to the walls so that inmates could use the springs to exercise while lying on their beds. After a flu epidemic that killed thousands, Joseph Pilates' fitness regimen was given credit for the fact that none of these inmates succumbed to the virus.

After the war, Pilates returned to Germany, settling in Hamburg where he continued with his fitness program, working with the local police force until he was drafted into the army. In 1926, disenchanted with Germany, he decided to set sail for the U.S. On board ship, he met a young nurse, Clara, who later became his wife.

Arriving in New York, he set up his first exercise studio at 939 Eighth Avenue. Little is known about the early years of the studio, but by the 1940s, he had achieved great popularity in the dance world. By the 1960s, many of New York's dancers were regular visitors to his studio, as were actors, gymnasts, and athletes. One of his more famous regulars was George Balanchine, who invited Joseph Pilates to instruct his ballerinas at the New York City Ballet. Since the 1960s, the Pilates method has continued to grow in popularity. In recent years, many more people have discovered the benefits of Pilates and this technique is becoming one of the most popular fitness systems.

The original exercises, devised by Joseph Pilates in the 1920s, consisted of thirty-four moves. Pilates' influences came from his studies of various sports and exercise routines from both Eastern and Western disciplines. His routine was not simply a set of physical movements separate from every other aspect of life, but part of a program of health care designed to improve an individual's overall fitness and well-being. Pilates never formalized his routine, instead adapting the moves to the needs of each individual. Consequently, many of his followers have developed their own version of the Pilates technique. The result of this is that, although the basic principles of Pilates are unchanging, the actual teachings now vary slightly in style and emphasis.

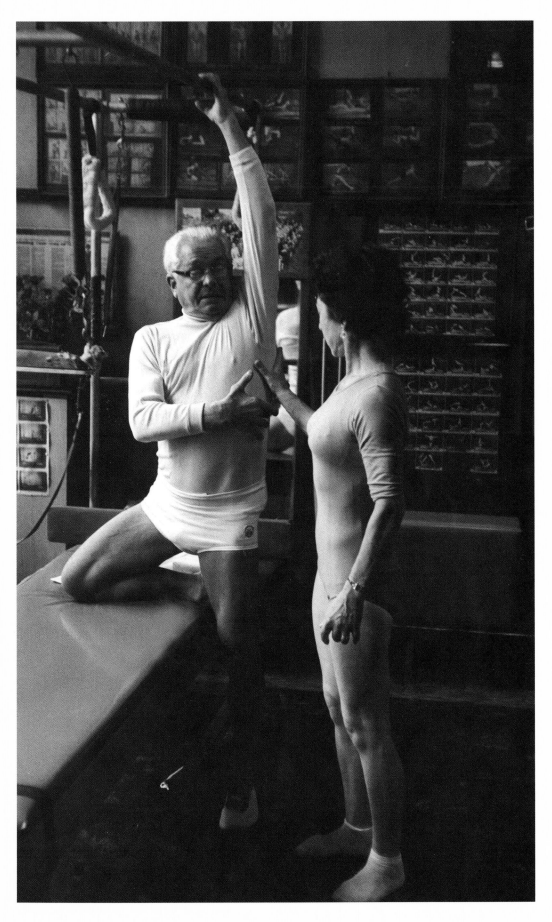

left: Joseph Pilates, at the age of eighty, in his New York studio, showing a pupil which muscle is engaging.

physiology

the skeleton

The skeleton can be classified into two separate parts:

1 The central, or axial, skeleton—head, thorax, and vertebral column

2 The extremities, or appendicular, skeleton—pelvis and bones of the upper and lower body

The functions of the skeleton are as follows:

- support for the body
- protection of internal organs
- movement, through muscle attachments onto bones
- manufacture of red and white blood cells
- storage of minerals, particularly calcium and phosphate

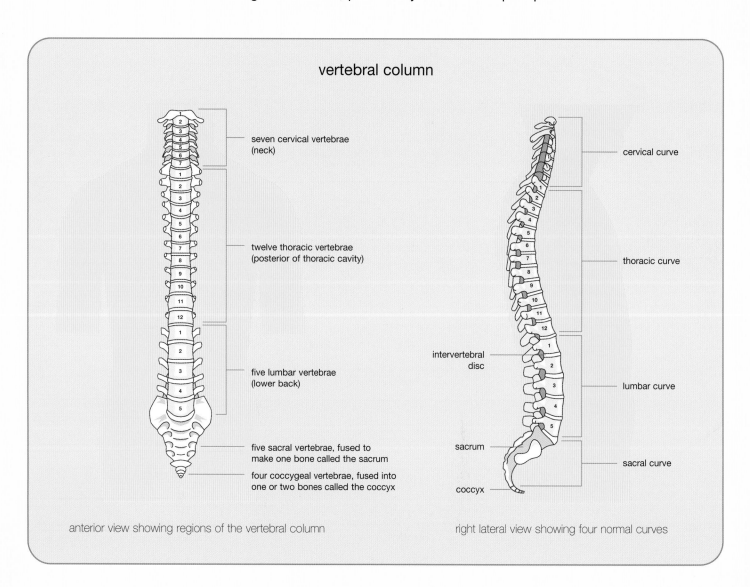

vertebral column

seven cervical vertebrae
(neck)

twelve thoracic vertebrae
(posterior of thoracic cavity)

five lumbar vertebrae
(lower back)

five sacral vertebrae, fused to
make one bone called the sacrum

four coccygeal vertebrae, fused into
one or two bones called the coccyx

intervertebral
disc

sacrum

coccyx

cervical curve

thoracic curve

lumbar curve

sacral curve

anterior view showing regions of the vertebral column

right lateral view showing four normal curves

the vertebral column

The vertebral column, along with the skull, ribs, and sternum, forms the axial skeleton.

The spine is a natural *S*-shape, with each of its bones separated by fibrocartilaginous intervertebral disks. It provides protection for the spinal cord and spinal nerve roots, support for the weight of the body, and helps to keep correct posture. The natural curves and the disks allow the spine to act in a springlike fashion, absorbing shock and making actions more agile. When the spinal curves are altered, stresses are placed on the spine that can lead to pain or bad posture, e.g., lower-back pain caused by long periods sitting at a desk.

The vertebral column is composed of thirty-three separate bones, or vertebrae, separated by intervertebral discs. They are made up of seven cervical vertebrae (neck), twelve thoracic vertebrae (posterior of thoracic cavity), five lumbar vertebrae (lower back), five sacral vertebrae, fused to make one bone called the sacrum, and four coccygeal vertebrae, fused into one or two bones called the coccyx (tailbone).

the muscles

There are three different types of muscle in the body:

- **Cardiac muscle**—found only in the heart.
- **Smooth (involuntary) muscle**—found in the gut and intestines, works without our conscious control to push food through the digestive system.
- **Striped/striated (voluntary) muscle**—muscles that attach to bones and contract and relax to create movement.

The central part of the muscle is composed of bundles of thin, parallel fibers, surrounded by connective tissue. A muscle fiber is served with a nerve ending, or motor end plate, which receives messages from the brain in order for the muscle to contract. Where gross motor movements occur, e.g., the large muscles of the thighs, one motor end plate will serve lots of muscle fibers. Where fine movements are needed, e.g., in the face or fingers, one motor end plate will serve only a few fibers. The strength of a muscular contraction depends on the number of fibers stimulated.

Muscles can only pull, not push, and so they work in opposing pairs to cause movements throughout the body. When one of the opposing pair contracts (shortens), the other must relax or stretch, and vice versa.

the stretch reflex

The stretch reflex is a protective mechanism within the muscle involving cells called muscle spindles. When a muscle is stretched too quickly, the muscle spindles react, causing the muscle to automatically contract to prevent tearing. To avoid this reflex reaction, always move into a stretch slowly and gradually.

technique principles

The essential principles of Pilates are:

- concentration
- breath
- centering
- control
- precision
- flowing movement
- isolation
- routine

concentration

Pilates is a technique that requires focus and concentration—it is not a form of mindless repetition in which your body runs on automatic and your mind switches off. Every movement is carefully controlled, and the mind needs to stay alert, allowing the mind and body to work together.

breath

Appropriate use of the breath is vital to correct performance of the Pilates exercises. Many people have a tendency to hold their breath while exercising or to take shallow breaths into the upper chest. This causes tension buildup in the body and inhibits the supply of oxygen to the muscles, reducing the performance of the muscles.

centering

The center referred to is also known as the abdominals, or central core, and even the "powerhouse." The Pilates system places its focus of power and control at the body's center of gravity (the area approximately two inches below the navel), with all moves being controlled by the contraction of the abdominal muscles. By working from this central core, we are able to stretch and lengthen the muscles without any risk of strain or injury to your spine and neck.

control

Muscle control is essential in order to maintain correct posture and alignment while working the muscles. In Pilates, we strengthen the body by working against gravity, using slow, controlled movements—the slower the movement, the stronger we become.

precision

Precise execution of the moves is one of the keys to the effectiveness of the Pilates technique and requires patience, practice, and concentration to achieve. To begin with, it can be very difficult to remember all the different points, but as you become more proficient, this will start to happen automatically and controlling the muscles while breathing, lengthening, and keeping your spine in a neutral position will eventually become second nature.

flowing movements

Pilates movements should be as smooth and even as possible. Each sequence should be repeated slowly, using a continuous, flowing movement that is at an even pace in time with the breathing.

isolation

To effectively execute the various Pilates moves, we need to develop an acute awareness of the different parts of our physical body so that we can practice the individual exercises in a precise, controlled manner, working one set of muscles while at the same time maintaining correct posture, breathing, and alignment and ensuring that any muscles that do not need to be involved stay relaxed.

routine

By developing routines and practicing regularly (even if only for a few minutes) we gradually improve our technique and enhance our skills and abilities.

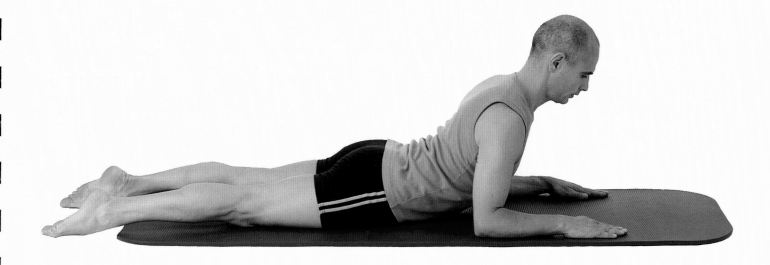

the pilates body

neutral spine

Neutral spine, also known as "the neutral position," or simply "neutral," is a fundamental part of the Pilates technique. Neutral is thought to be the natural position for the spine. Exercising with the spine in this position allows us to use the body as originally intended, improving our posture and balance and developing our strength, mobility, and muscle control, increasing our efficiency as we perform everyday activities and reducing our risk of back injury or deterioration of posture.

finding neutral

In order to benefit fully from the Pilates exercises, it is important to develop the ability to maintain neutral spine while standing, sitting, or lying down.

finding neutral while sitting

❶ Sit on the edge of a chair with your feet hip-width apart, feet flat on the floor, and your hands resting lightly on your thighs. Round your back slightly, tilting your pelvis forward and flattening out your back or rounding it slightly.

❷ Now tilt your pelvis backward, creating an exaggerated arch in your lower back.

❸ Move between these points until you find the halfway position with your back straight, but with a slight natural curve in your lower back. This is the neutral position.

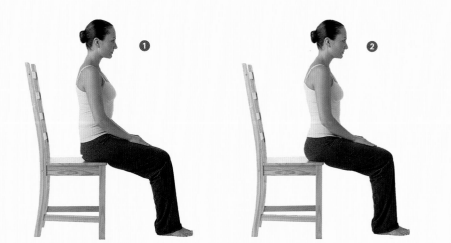

VARIATION

To find neutral while lying down, lie on your back with your feet hip-width apart, knees pointing to the ceiling, and arms resting by your sides with the palms facing downward, then follow the instructions given on the previous page. Once you have found neutral spine in this position, there should be a slight gap between your waist and the floor—just enough for you to slide your hand under your lower back. When exercising lying on your front (in the prone position), your feet are usually parallel. If you find this to be uncomfortable, are unable to hold this position, or it causes tension in your legs and buttocks, then bring the big toes together and drop your heels out to the side. Over time, as your flexibility improves, you will be able to lie on your front with your feet parallel.

the sitting position

In Pilates, many of the exercises begin with you sitting on the floor, either with knees bent or legs stretched out in front of you. Even in this position, it is essential that you are able to find neutral spine before you begin the move.

❶ The posture illustrated is incorrect—when sitting with legs outstretched, keep the knees soft and feel your buttocks in contact with the floor. Avoid tilting the pelvis forward and leaning back too far, creating unnecessary tension in the upper back, the front of the body, and the neck.

❷ This raised knee posture is not being held correctly. Here the front of the body is collapsed and the lower back unsupported, with the pelvis tilting too far forward. The shoulders are slouched and there is tension in the lower back and neck.

❸ In this version, we have the opposite problem—the pelvis is tilted too far back and there is tension in the back and neck from attempting to hold it too straight.

❹ This picture shows the correct sitting position: sitting upright, lengthening through the spine and along the back of the neck, while retaining the natural curve of the spine and contracting the abdominals. It is shown here with legs outstretched; the same body position would also be used when sitting with knees raised.

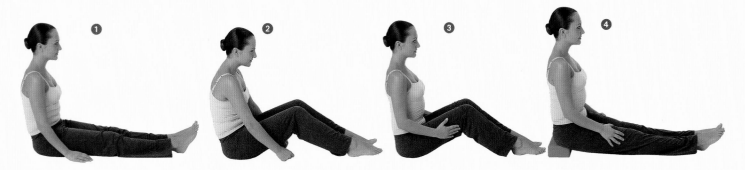

posture and breathing

standing in neutral

Healthy posture is essential to Pilates. We need to educate our bodies so that we can stand symmetrically, with the spine in alignment, our weight evenly distributed over both feet, and the central core supporting the body.

❶ Stand with your feet in parallel, hip-width apart, knees soft, arms resting by your sides, shoulders dropped. Check that your weight is evenly distributed over both feet and between the front and the back of each foot. Your knees should be directly over your ankles. Make sure that your head is balanced correctly on top of your spine. Avoid jutting your chin forward. Draw the shoulder blades down and back behind you. Lengthen up through your spine and neck; imagine a thread running through the body, out of the top of your head and out through your tailbone down to the floor. Relax your shoulders, dropping them downward without rounding them forward or forcing them back

❷ Here the posture is held incorrectly—the back has been flattened out, creating tension in the spine and neck.

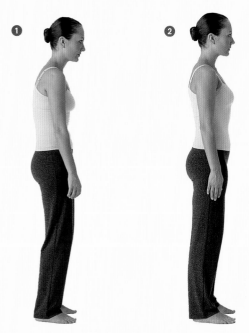

contracting the abdominals

In the Pilates technique, great importance is given to supporting and controlling the movements with the abdominal core. In order to achieve this, we pull up on the muscles of the pelvic floor (as if we were interrupting a flow of urine), while at the same time pulling the abdominal muscles back toward your spine. As we do this, we need to avoid rounding out our lumbar spine, keeping the back in neutral position. This is sometimes referred to as "navel to spine."

breathing

Correct breathing increases the efficiency of the oxygen supply to the muscles. For this, we focus on the lower part of the rib cage and the abdominal muscles. Using these muscles, we expand the lungs outward (laterally), rather than lifting them upward, bringing air right to the bottom of the lungs. This increases the efficiency of the oxygen supply to the muscles. In order to coordinate the movements with the breathing, we need to establish rhythm. As a general rule, we inhale as we prepare and exhale as we stretch or move.

❶ Stand on the floor, feet parallel and hip-width apart, your weight centered and evenly distributed between both feet. Place your hands at the base of your ribs with your middle fingers touching. Check that your spine is in neutral and your spine and neck lengthened. Drop your shoulders and draw the shoulder blades back and down.

❷ Focusing on moving the lower part of the chest and keeping the upper part relaxed, inhale and as you take breath into your lungs, imagine that your rib cage is stretching out to the sides. Avoid raising your shoulders as you breathe. Your back will expand and your hands and fingers will separate. Exhale, allowing the back and rib cage to contract and the hands to return to the starting position. Repeat several times, but avoid hyperventilating.

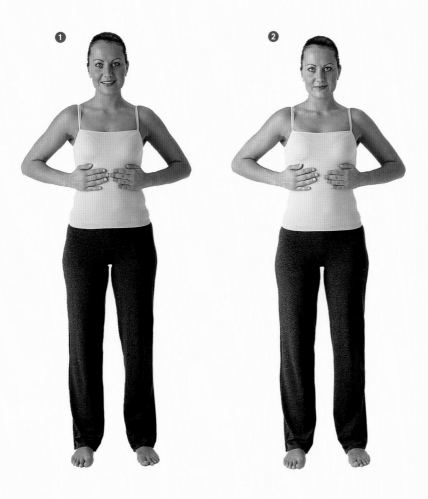

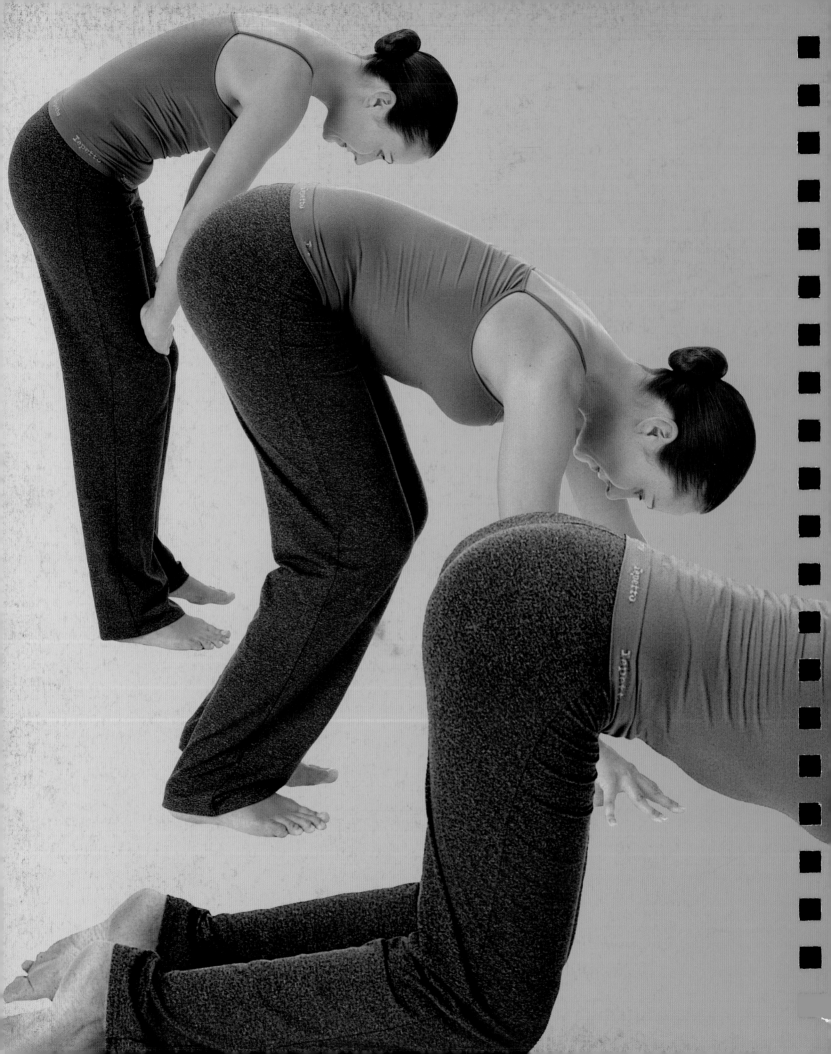

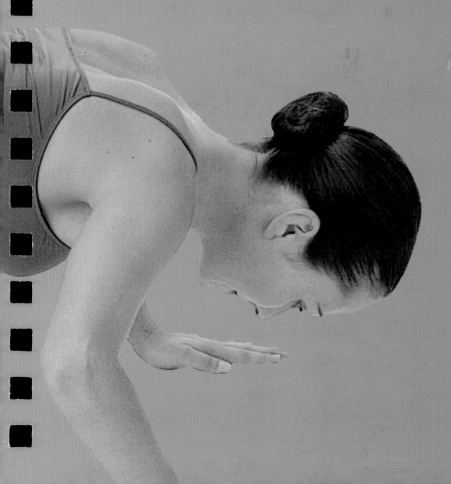

part 2

the movements

warm-ups

Warming up is an essential part of any exercise routine and should never be skipped or avoided. It improves the circulation to the muscles and gently prepares your body for the movements ahead. The best way to begin is by spending a minute or two practicing your breathing. As you do so, put aside the events of the day, along with any

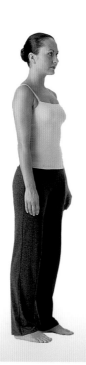
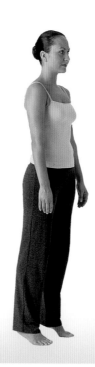
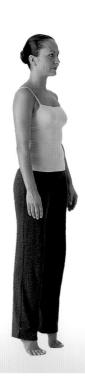

balance

This movement gives your body a gentle stretch and improves your balance, while warming up the muscles of your legs and feet.

❶ Stand in neutral, with your feet slightly apart, knees soft. Focus straight ahead, lengthening along your spine and neck as you do so. Drop your shoulders and draw the shoulder blades back and down behind you. Relax the arms. Inhale.

❷ Exhale, contract your abdominals, and keep lengthening up through your spine, allowing your heels to raise off the ground.

Think of the crown of your head lifting straight up toward the ceiling and your tailbone releasing down to the floor. Keep looking straight ahead to help you balance.

❸ Continue to exhale as you slowly and smoothly roll up through your feet onto your toes. Keep your ankles and feet in parallel—avoid letting your ankles open out to the sides. Inhale, lengthening your spine as much as you can. Exhale, contract your abdominals, and slowly roll back down through the feet, continually lengthening up through your spine as you do so. Repeat five to ten times.

worries you may have, and focus your attention on your body, letting go of any tension that you may be holding. Find your neutral position (see pages 22–23) and lengthen along your spine and the back of your neck.

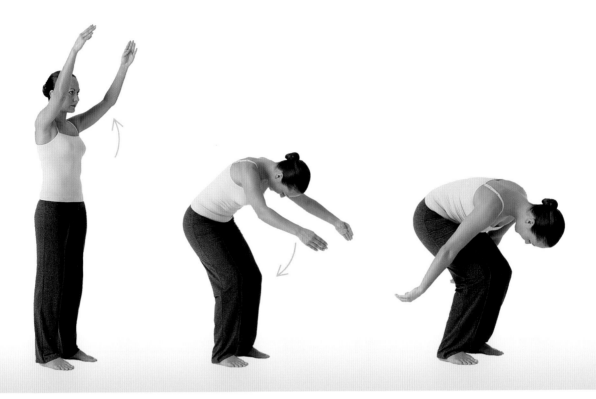

arm swings

This arm-swing movement stimulates the circulation and warms up your spine and back muscles. The move should be slow, smooth, and controlled.

❶ Stand with your feet parallel and your back in neutral. Lengthen along your spine and neck, then inhale and raise your arms up toward the ceiling.

❷ Exhale, contract your abdominals, and swing your arms downward, curving over with your spine, relaxing your head and shoulders, and bending your knees.

❸ Still exhaling, continue with the swinging motion, taking your arms back behind you. Inhale as you slowly swing your arms and roll back up to standing. Repeat five to ten times, lengthening your spine up toward the ceiling a little more each time you roll back up.

warm-ups continued

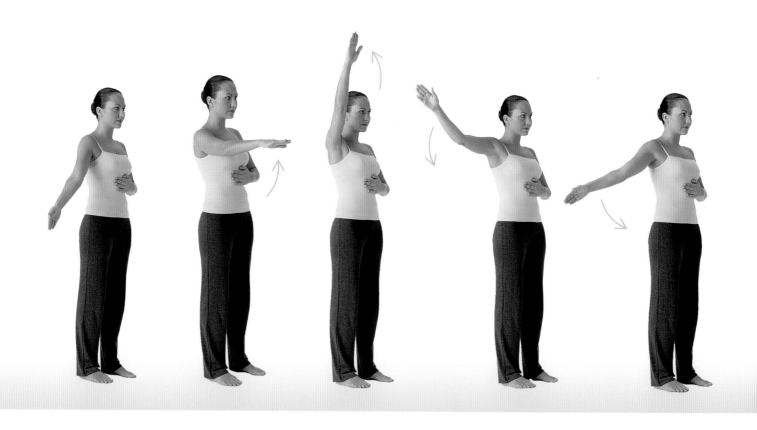

single arm circles

This exercise opens up your shoulders, gently stretches across the chest, and releases tension in your neck and shoulder area. Make sure you work both arms evenly.

❶ Stand with your feet in parallel, slightly apart. Place your left hand on your rib cage to monitor your breathing. Inhale and raise your right arm in front of you, slightly to the side.

❷ Exhale, contract your abdominals, and start to circle your arm forward, keeping your shoulders level and fingers

lengthened. If you are finding it difficult to circle your arm without raising your shoulder, move your arm further away from your body and make the circles smaller.

❸ Continue the movement, circling your arm up, then slightly behind you, and back down. Keep the eyes focused forward. Circle your right arm ten times on one side, then switch and do the same for your left arm. Maintain a slow, steady movement in time with your breathing.

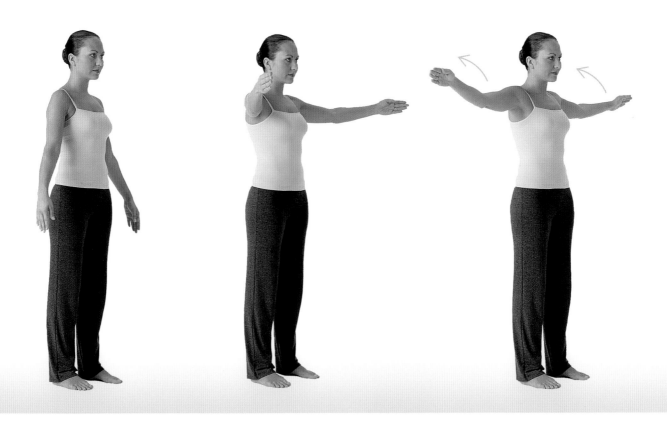

double arm circles

This movement is an intensified version of the single arm circles, stimulating the circulation, mobilizing your shoulders and your arms, and opening out your chest. Focus on keeping your abdominals contracted and your back in neutral as you carry out this exercise.

1 Stand with your feet parallel, slightly apart, knees soft. Focus your eyes straight in front of you. Inhale and lengthen up through your spine and neck. Keeping your shoulders relaxed and down, raise your arms out to the sides slightly.

2 Exhale, contract your abdominals, and start to circle the arms out to the sides and up, lengthening your arms out from your shoulders and keeping your fingers long.

3 Inhale as you take your arms back, around, and down to complete the circle. Keep the movement slow and continuous, taking your arms to just above shoulder height at the top of the circle and slightly behind you at the back. If you have difficulty keeping the alignment while circling your arms, make smaller circles. Do ten circles in one direction, then ten circles in the other. Make sure you work both arms evenly, particularly if one side feels weaker than the other.

push-up

beginner

This exercise helps to strengthen your abdominals, lower back, and upper body. It is a continuous flowing movement that should be done as slowly as possible, using a controlled movement. Keep your lower abdominals contracted to focus the strengthening effect of the move and provide support for your lower back.

❶ Stand in neutral with your feet hip-width apart and your knees soft (slightly bent). Inhale and contract your lower abdominals. Avoid hunching your shoulders or lifting your chest.

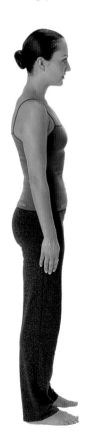

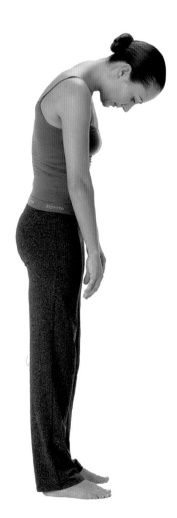

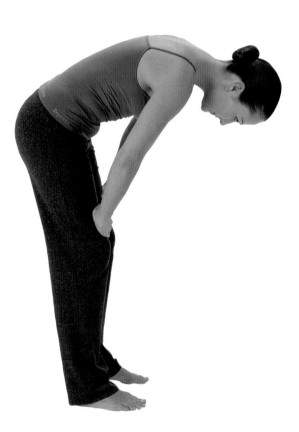

❷ Exhale, drop your head forward, and start to roll down toward the floor, using a slow, controlled movement.

❸ Continue to roll down as you exhale. If you run out of breath, stop and inhale, then exhale and continue to roll the rest of the way down. Think of curling your spine downward one vertebrae at a time, starting at the top and working down to your tailbone. Keep your knees soft (slightly bent) and your arms relaxed throughout this movement, and avoid sticking your tailbone out. As you keep curling down toward the floor, allow your hands to slide gently onto your knees.

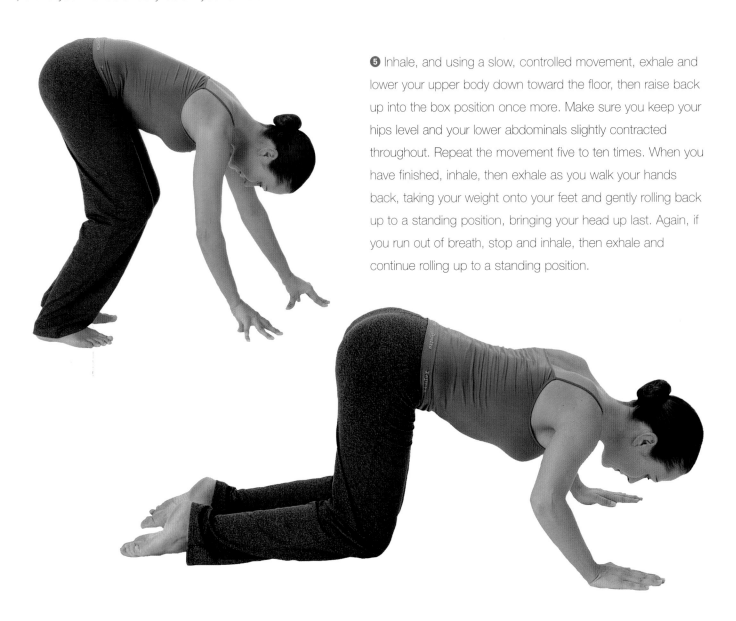

❹ When you have rolled down as far as you comfortably can, bend your knees and drop your hands, fingertips first, onto the floor. Keeping your eyes focused straight down, inhale, and, as you exhale, walk your hands forward, away from your body, gently dropping onto your knees so that you are now on all fours in the box position with your knees directly below your hips and your hands directly below your shoulders.

❺ Inhale, and using a slow, controlled movement, exhale and lower your upper body down toward the floor, then raise back up into the box position once more. Make sure you keep your hips level and your lower abdominals slightly contracted throughout. Repeat the movement five to ten times. When you have finished, inhale, then exhale as you walk your hands back, taking your weight onto your feet and gently rolling back up to a standing position, bringing your head up last. Again, if you run out of breath, stop and inhale, then exhale and continue rolling up to a standing position.

swimming (prone)

In this exercise, the aim is to lengthen down through your arms and legs, releasing your arms away from your shoulders and your legs away from your hips. Beware of lifting the limbs too high. Keep them low and parallel to the ground. Your hips should remain level and in contact with the floor, and your body should stay still throughout, with your spine lengthened and the lower abdominal muscles contracted. Your legs and arms should work in isolation, lengthening and stretching away from your body. If you feel discomfort in your neck or lower back, stop.

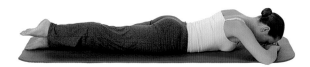

❶ Lie facedown in the prone position with your forehead resting on your arms, keeping your shoulders relaxed and lengthening out through the back of your neck. Find neutral and then breathe in, contract the abdominal muscles slightly,

and lengthen down through your right leg, sliding it along the floor and then allowing it to rise very slightly off the ground. Keep your buttocks relaxed. Breathe out and lower your right leg and do the same on the other side. Repeat ten times.

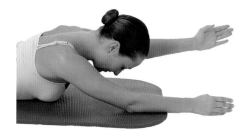

❷ Reach both arms out in front of you along the floor, palms facing. Relax your shoulders, lengthen the back of your neck, and focus your eyes straight down to the floor. Contract your abdominal muscles slightly and breathe in. Breathe out as you lift and lengthen your right arm and your left leg simultaneously. Breathe in and relax as you lower back down to the floor.

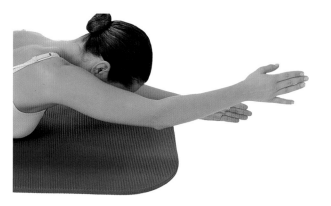

❸ Do exactly the same for your left arm and right leg, again starting by sliding the arms and legs along the floor and then raising them very slightly off the ground.

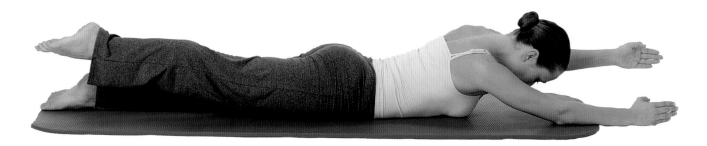

❹ Repeat ten times on each side.

swimming (kneeling)

Once you have mastered the Swimming (prone) exercise you are ready to move on to this variation. Swimming (kneeling) is a development of the previous exercise, and it is best to always begin with some repetitions of Swimming (prone) before attempting this variation.

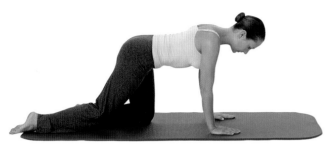

① Kneel in the box position—on all fours with your knees directly below your hips and your hands directly below your shoulders. Keep your eyes focused down to the floor and your back and neck lengthened. Breathe in. Contract your lower abdominals slightly and allow your right leg to slide back along the ground, away from your body, then raise it off the ground. Make sure your leg remains parallel to your body (don't let it swing out) and keep the hips level. Repeat for your left leg.

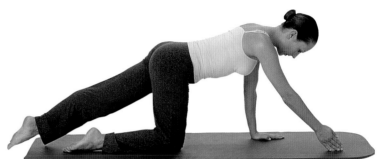

② When you are ready, you can add the arms, working your arms and legs in opposition, as before, and lengthening out through your arm, hand, and fingers to the wall in front of you and down through your leg to the wall behind. Inhale as you lower your arm and leg, and exhale as you lift and lengthen. Your arm should rise until it is just in front of your face, while your leg rises until it is level with the rest of your body. Beware of raising your leg too high, as this will force your hips out of the correct alignment for this exercise.

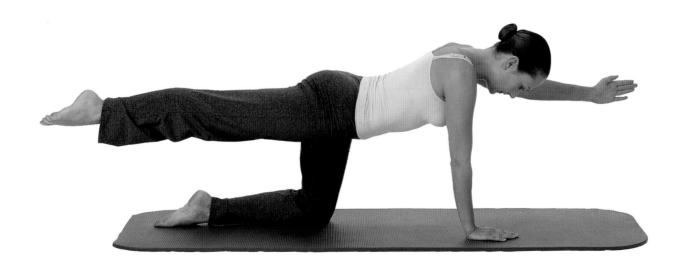

③ Repeat the exercise ten times on each side.

the plank

beginner/intermediate

This exercise works to strengthen your abdominals, lower back, upper body, legs, and arms, and improves balance and core stability. Keep your hips level and your spine and the back of your neck lengthened as you raise up off the ground.

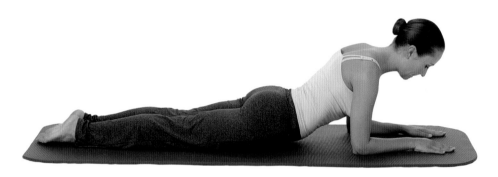

❶ Position yourself facedown with your forearms resting on the floor. Focus your eyes down on the floor in front of you and think of bringing your shoulders down your back and allowing your spine to lengthen. Inhale and contract your lower abdominals.

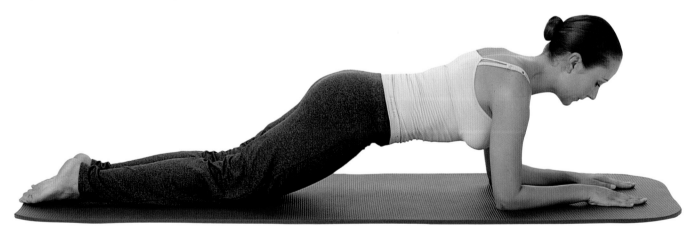

❷ Exhale and raise yourself gently up onto your knees, keeping your focus downward and your spine and neck lengthened.

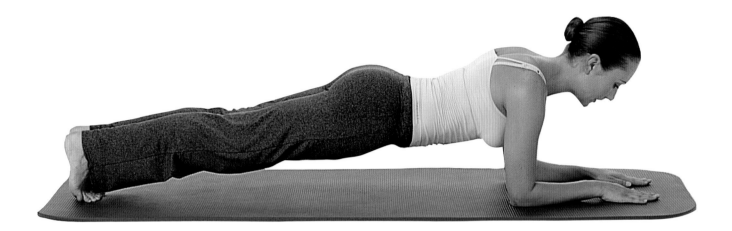

❸ Inhale, tucking your toes under and contracting the lower abdominals. Keeping your legs straight and your spine lengthened, exhale and push up off the ground. Make sure you keep your shoulders pulled down toward your back and your elbows soft. Keep your body in a line, parallel to the floor. Inhale, and exhale as you lower yourself back down to the floor. Repeat five to ten times.

VARIATION: advanced

Once you have mastered the above exercise and developed sufficient strength and stability in your abdominals, back, arms, and legs, you are ready to try this challenging variation: Position yourself as for Step 1, but this time with your hands directly below your shoulders and your toes tucked under. As you raise yourself off the ground, lift your knees and straighten your arms (keeping your elbows soft). Your neck, back, and legs should be in a straight line—like a plank.

the roll up

beginner/intermediate

This is an excellent exercise for strengthening the abdominal muscles and mobilizing and strengthening the back. Concentrate on making your movement as flowing as possible, making sure it is slow and controlled throughout. This exercise is not meant to be a struggle. Keep your abdominals tucked in and avoid making any jerky movements. Think about rolling back vertebra by vertebra, starting at the base of your spine and imagining the lower back opening and releasing as you roll down to the floor. Keep your knees bent and your feet firmly on the floor.

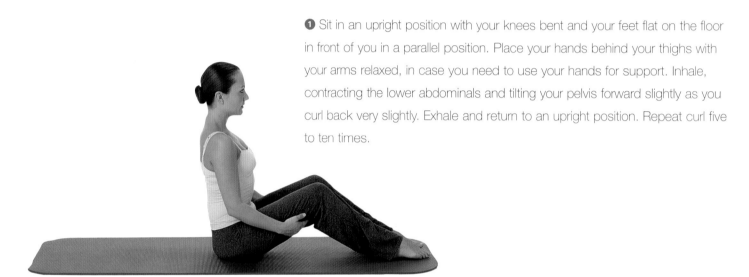

❶ Sit in an upright position with your knees bent and your feet flat on the floor in front of you in a parallel position. Place your hands behind your thighs with your arms relaxed, in case you need to use your hands for support. Inhale, contracting the lower abdominals and tilting your pelvis forward slightly as you curl back very slightly. Exhale and return to an upright position. Repeat curl five to ten times.

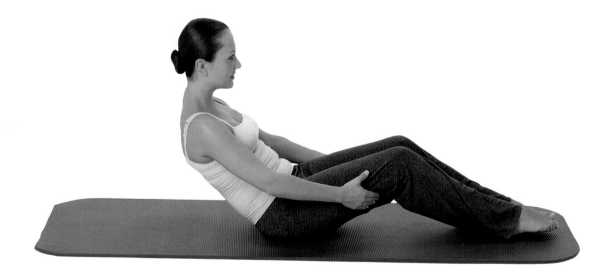

❷ Gradually increase the range of movement backward and forward, this time inhaling as you contract and exhaling as you curl back, then inhaling at your furthest point and exhaling as you return to upright. Keep your focus straight ahead in front of you. Use your hands to help you, if you need to; otherwise let go of your thighs and place your hands by your sides, palms facing upward.

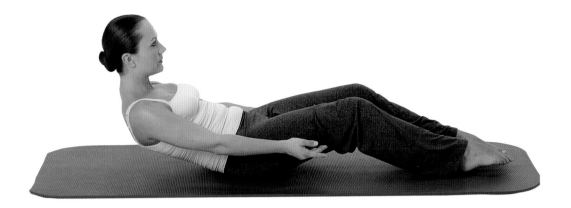

❸ As your abdominal strength improves and your flexibility increases, you will be able to curl further down toward the floor. If you can, then roll all the way down to the floor, keeping your focus straight ahead in front of you for as long as possible.

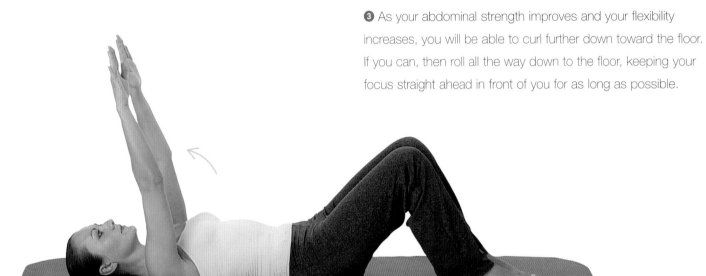

❹ As you lie back on the mat with your knees bent, allow your arms to come straight up, parallel to your body and back behind you, level with your face. Inhale, check that your abdominals are contracted, exhale, bring your arms back, keeping your elbows soft, and then tuck your chin into your chest slightly and roll back to the upright position. Use your abdominal muscles to pull you up, there should be no discomfort in your neck and shoulders. Repeat five to ten times.

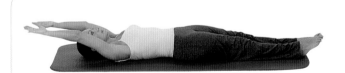

VARIATION: intermediate/advanced

Once you have mastered the above exercise, an alternative to Step 4 is to allow your legs to stretch out along the ground as you take your arms back behind your head. When rolling back up, return your legs to a bent position at the same time as you bring your arms back toward your body. A further development would be to have your legs straight out in front of you, but only attempt this if you have a great deal of flexibility in the lower back and strength in your abdominals.

rolling back

beginner/intermediate/advanced

This exercise strengthens your abdominals and opens out your lower back. Keep your knees tucked in toward your chest and allow the momentum of the movement, along with your abdominal muscles, to bring you back to a sitting position. If your lower back is stiff or tight, your neck is painful or sore, or you have any difficulty at all with this exercise, go easy on yourself—leave it for a while and focus on the Roll Up exercise instead until your strength and flexibility has improved and you can try again.

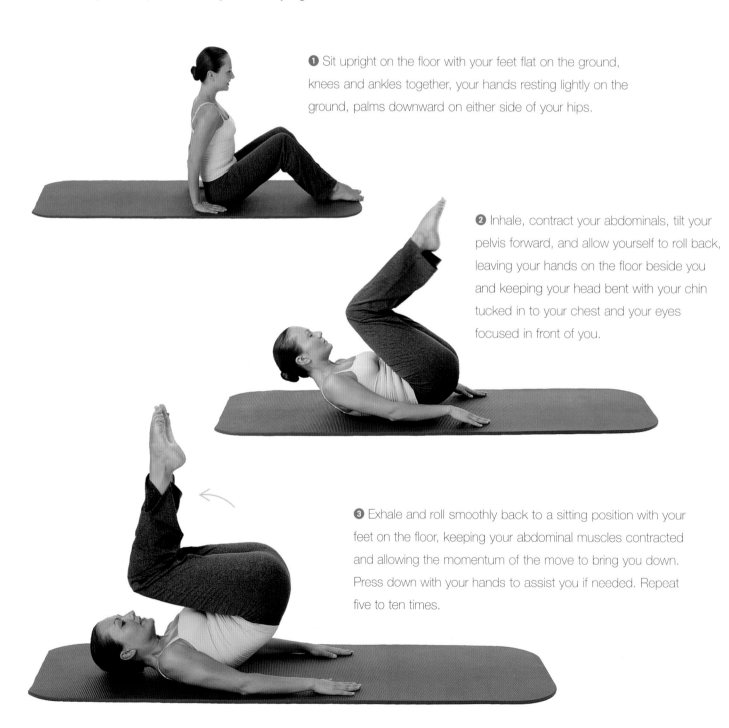

❶ Sit upright on the floor with your feet flat on the ground, knees and ankles together, your hands resting lightly on the ground, palms downward on either side of your hips.

❷ Inhale, contract your abdominals, tilt your pelvis forward, and allow yourself to roll back, leaving your hands on the floor beside you and keeping your head bent with your chin tucked in to your chest and your eyes focused in front of you.

❸ Exhale and roll smoothly back to a sitting position with your feet on the floor, keeping your abdominal muscles contracted and allowing the momentum of the move to bring you down. Press down with your hands to assist you if needed. Repeat five to ten times.

❹ If you do not need your hands to help you, rest them on your shins and keep them in this position throughout. Try controlling the movement even more and slowing it down to intensify the exercise.

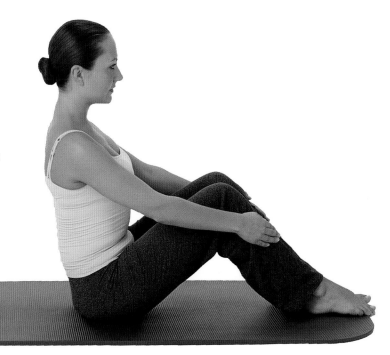

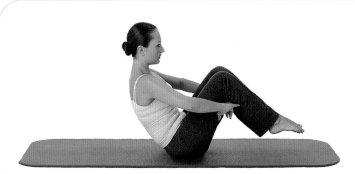

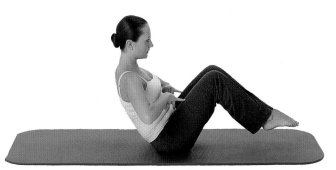

TIP 1

The correct leg position for this exercise is to have your knees at a slight angle—use the thumb and little finger of one hand as a guide. Focus on maintaining a consistent amount of space behind your knee as you carry out this exercise.

TIP 2

Again, use your thumb and little finger as a measure to check that you have the correct amount of space between your thighs and your ribs. Keep this gap consistent as you roll to ensure that your legs are held at the correct angle.

the hundred

beginner

This is the exercise that Joseph Pilates used as his initial warm-up exercise. The movement focuses primarily on working the abdominal core while keeping your spine in neutral and is excellent for improving muscle control. There are several variations of this movement, with increasing levels of difficulty. Avoid feeling pressured to advance too quickly through these variations. You will get much more benefit from working a less demanding option while maintaining the correct alignment than by overstretching yourself and struggling with the exercise.

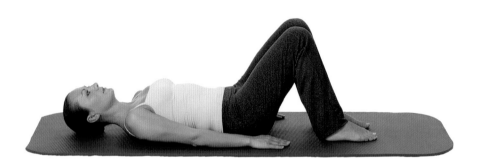

❶ Lie on the floor with your legs bent, knees pointing up to the ceiling, feet parallel, and your arms by your sides with palms facing downward. Your spine should be in neutral with a small gap between your waist and the floor—just enough for you to slide your hand under your lower back.

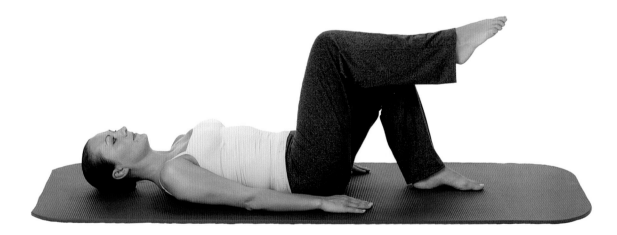

❷ Keeping your spine in neutral with your hips relaxed and your eyes focused up toward the ceiling, inhale, then as you exhale, contract your abdominals slightly and lift your right leg until the shin is parallel to the floor, with the knee at a right angle. Holding your legs in this position, drop your shoulders and lengthen your arms, lifting and lowering with a pulsing action, five times as you inhale and five times as you exhale, until you reach one hundred. Squeeze your ankles together as you pulse your arms, and keep your eyes focused up toward the ceiling.

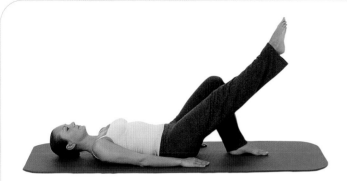

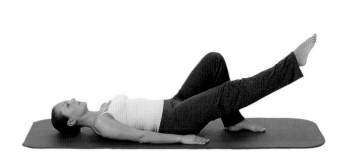

VARIATION 1: beginner/intermediate

If your abdominal muscles are reasonably strong, you might want to try this variation. As you exhale, extend your leg, lowering it slightly and lengthening away from the hip, down your leg, and out through the foot. Check that your spine is still in neutral with your abdominals contracted slightly. Pulse the arms as described in Step 2, to a count of fifty. Repeat for the other leg.

VARIATION 2: intermediate/advanced

To give yourself a greater challenge and increase the intensity of the exercise in the abdominal area, exhale and lower the extended leg a few inches further down toward the floor. Pulse your arms as in Step 2, then inhale and return your leg to the right-angle position. Exhale and lower it back down to the floor. Repeat for the other leg.

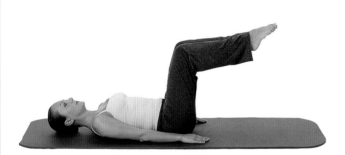

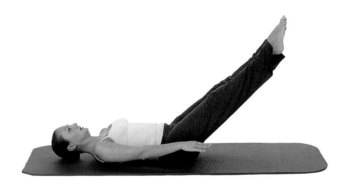

VARIATION 3: intermediate/advanced

For a further development of this exercise, adopt the position described in Step 1, then inhale and gently release your lower back toward the floor (this is called "imprinting"). Keep your buttocks relaxed, contract your lower abdominals slightly, and exhale, lifting your right leg until the shin is parallel to the floor with the knees at a right angle. Inhale, and as you exhale, raise the other leg, too. Pulse your arms as for Step 2, then inhale, and as you exhale, lower the first leg back down to the floor, then inhale, and as you exhale, lower the other leg.

VARIATION 4: advanced

Once you have improved your strength and stability, you are ready for this variation of the Hundred. Follow Variation 3, then once you have achieved the right-angle position with both your legs, inhale, exhale, and extend both legs out, lowering them a little toward the floor if you can. Think of squeezing the inner thighs together as you do this part of the exercise. Lengthen through the back of your neck, drop the chin onto the chest, and raise your head away from the floor. Pulse your arms, then inhale, and as you exhale, return your legs to the right-angle position. Inhale, exhale, and lower the first leg back down to the floor, then inhale, and as you exhale, lower the other leg. Repeat five to ten times.

the seal

intermediate/advanced

This is a challenging move for some people; do not attempt it until you have mastered the basic levels of the Rolling Back move. For those who are able to attempt this exercise, it is particularly good for strengthening the abdominal core and improving balance and muscle control. If you feel any discomfort while doing this exercise, stop and return to the Rolling Back exercise to build up your strength and flexibility.

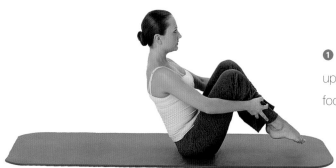

❶ Sit upright on the floor, as for the Rolling Back, lengthening up through your spine and back of your neck, with your eyes focused straight ahead.

❷ Rest your hands lightly on the front of the shins, inhale, contract your abdominals, and bring your feet off the floor, finding your point of balance. Draw the shoulder blades down your back and keep your shoulders relaxed and your neck lengthened.

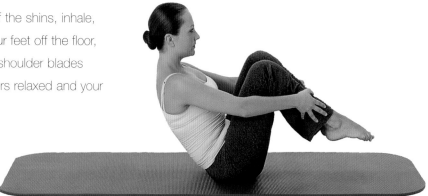

❸ Exhale, drop your head forward slightly, and start to roll back, your spine making contact with the floor, vertebra by vertebra, using a slow, flowing movement.

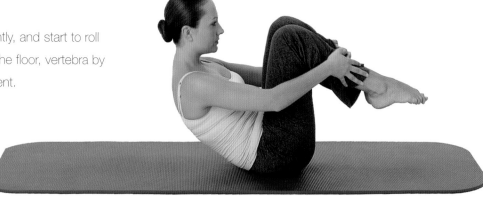

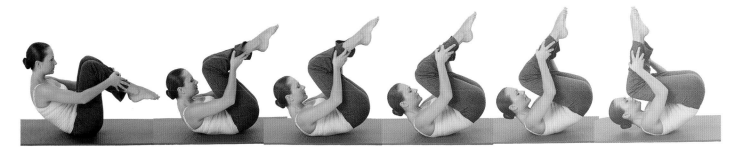

④ Continue to roll back onto the floor as you exhale, keeping your abdominals contracted and your eyes focused in front of you.

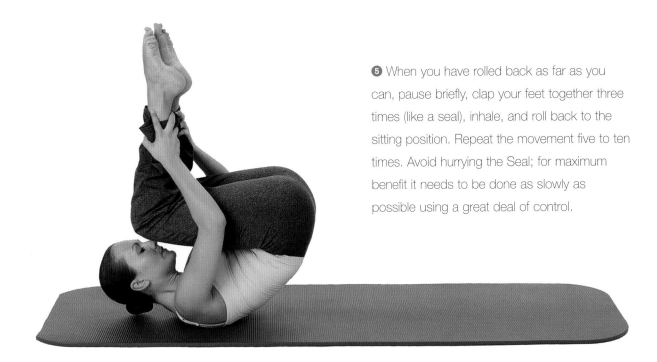

⑤ When you have rolled back as far as you can, pause briefly, clap your feet together three times (like a seal), inhale, and roll back to the sitting position. Repeat the movement five to ten times. Avoid hurrying the Seal; for maximum benefit it needs to be done as slowly as possible using a great deal of control.

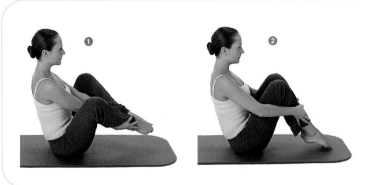

VARIATION: beginner/advanced

There are two possible hand positions for the Seal. You can either rest your hands on the front of your shins, just above your ankles (2), or try the slightly more difficult option of placing your hands between your legs and holding onto the backs of your ankles (1). Do not attempt this variation if it is at all uncomfortable for you.

spine stretch

beginner

This spine stretch is excellent for improving the mobility of the back. It has the added effect of stretching out the hamstrings at the back of your legs. Ideally, you should keep your legs as straight as possible throughout this movement, but avoid locking your knees.

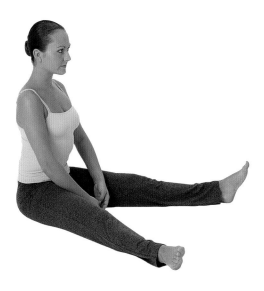

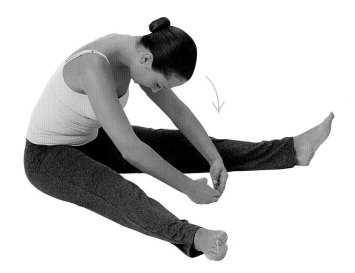

❶ Sit in an upright position with your back and neck lengthened and your legs slightly apart. Place your hands between your legs in a relaxed position. Inhale and contract your abdominals, tilting the pelvis forward slightly.

❷ Bend your head slightly in toward your chest, curve your upper back, and as you exhale, stretch forward toward your feet, allowing your arms to release forward at the same time. The action is one of stretching forward and down with the chest, one vertebrae at a time, avoiding collapsing your ribs at the front of your body—think of curving the upper body over a large beach ball.

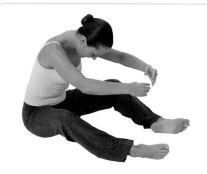

VARIATION

If your hamstrings are tight and the above version is uncomfortable or painful in any way, do the same exercise as described above, but use this position instead. Allow your legs to bend a little, with your knees dropped out to the side and the soles of your feet facing. The crucial element is for you to allow your upper back to rotate as much as possible, giving it the maximum opportunity to stretch out your upper spine.

the saw

beginner/intermediate

This stretch mobilizes the upper back, improving flexibility and helping to release any tension that is held here. As you stretch, think of your spine and neck lengthening. Avoid collapsing your upper body as you reach forward with your arm—imagine that you are reaching up and over a large beach ball.

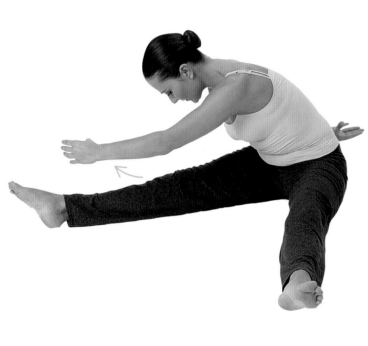

❶ Sit in an upright position with your legs apart at an angle of approximately forty-five degrees. Draw your shoulder blades back, then inhale, contract your lower abdominals, and tilt your pelvis forward slightly. At the same time, raise your arms to slightly below shoulder height, at the same angle as your legs, keeping your elbows soft. Exhale and reach your left arm forward over your right leg toward your foot, taking your right arm back behind you and twisting your upper body a little to the right, following the movement of your left arm. Make sure you keep your hips still and your legs and feet relaxed. It is only your abdominals and upper body that should be working.

❷ Inhale and return to center, then exhale and reach your right arm toward the left foot. Inhale and return to center. Repeat five to ten times on each side.

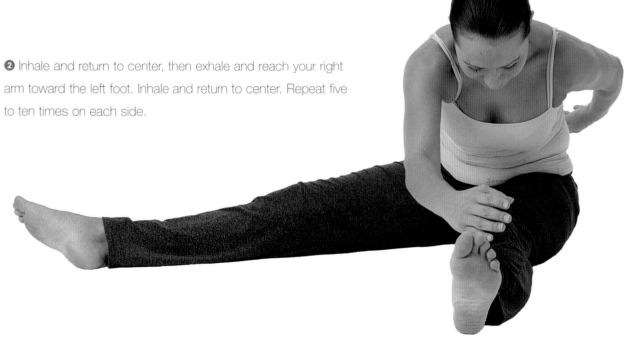

spine twist

beginner/intermediate

This spine rotation exercise improves the mobility in your mid- and upper back, helping to reduce any tension and stiffness. It is important for you to sit upright throughout this movement, keeping your spine lengthened. The movement should be a smooth, flowing twist at a steady pace in time with your breathing.

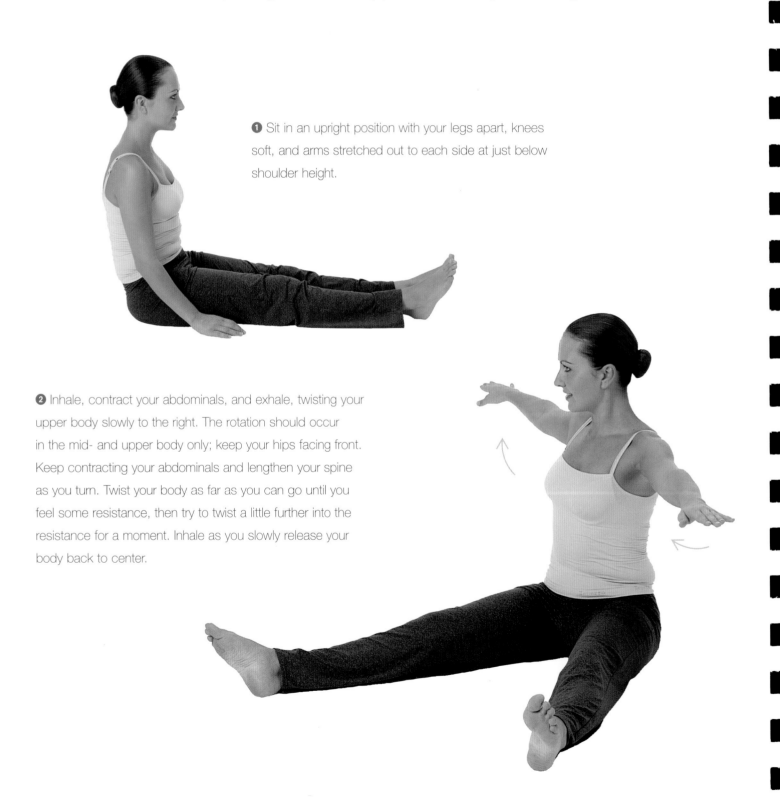

❶ Sit in an upright position with your legs apart, knees soft, and arms stretched out to each side at just below shoulder height.

❷ Inhale, contract your abdominals, and exhale, twisting your upper body slowly to the right. The rotation should occur in the mid- and upper body only; keep your hips facing front. Keep contracting your abdominals and lengthen your spine as you turn. Twist your body as far as you can go until you feel some resistance, then try to twist a little further into the resistance for a moment. Inhale as you slowly release your body back to center.

❸ Repeat Step 2, this time twisting around to the left. Remember to keep your arms and head in line with your body throughout the entire movement. Repeat the twist a total of five to ten times.

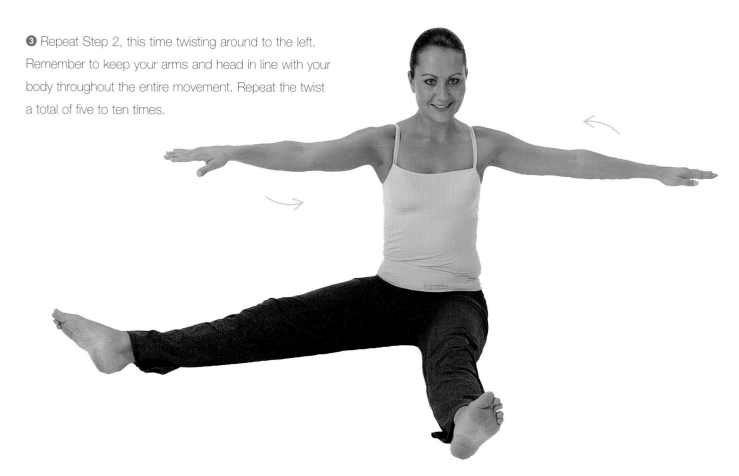

VARIATION: beginner/intermediate

This exercise is intended purely as a rotation exercise to mobilize your spine. If you are feeling tension and discomfort in your arms, shoulders, or hamstrings, or are finding it difficult to sit upright with your arms straight out in front of you, choose from these alternative arm and leg positions instead.

There are two other arm positions to choose from, both of which reduce the risk of tension in your shoulders and upper arms. Either fold your arms in front of you in a box position, palms facing downward, the fingertips of one hand touching the opposite elbow (option 1), or hands held together in front of you at breastbone height, fingertips touching, hands and arms relaxed (option 2).

As an alternative to sitting with your legs straight out in front of you, try sitting with legs crossed (option 1), or with legs bent and knees dropped to the sides, soles of the feet together (option 2).

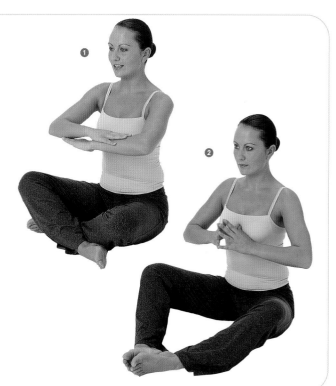

leg pull (prone)

intermediate/advanced

This exercise works to strengthen your abdominals, lower back, upper body, legs, and arms and improves balance and stability. Keep the hips level and your spine and the back of your neck lengthened throughout this exercise. If you prefer a less intense stretch, you can do your leg raises holding the positions shown in Step 1 and Step 2.

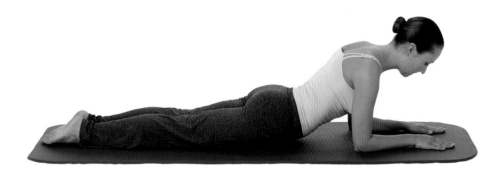

❶ Position yourself facedown with your forearms resting on the floor. Focus your eyes down on the floor in front of you and think of bringing your shoulders down your back and allowing your spine to lengthen. Inhale and contract your lower abdominals.

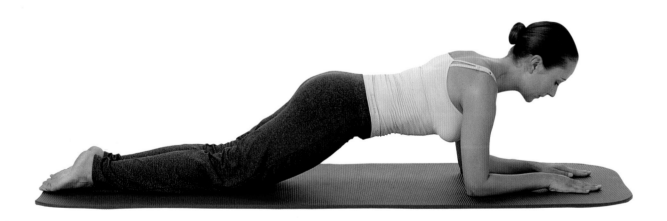

❷ Exhale and raise yourself gently up onto your knees, keeping your focus downward and your spine and neck lengthened. Inhale, tucking your toes under and contracting your lower abdominals. Keeping your legs straight and your spine lengthened, exhale and push up off the ground, leaving your forearms on the ground. Make sure you keep your shoulders pulled down toward your back and your elbows soft. Keep your body in a line, parallel to the floor. Avoid raising your bottom higher than your shoulders or letting it drop.

❹ Raise yourself up onto your hands, straightening your arms.
Check that you are still contracting your lower abdominals.
Make sure you keep your shoulders pulled back and your
elbows soft. Inhale.

❺ As you exhale, raise your left leg straight up behind, lengthening it away from your
body and keeping your hips level and your body in a line. Inhale as you lower your leg
and exhale as you raise it once more. Repeat for a total of five to ten leg raises, then
switch and do the same number of raises for the other leg. Inhale. Exhale as you lower
yourself back down to the ground.

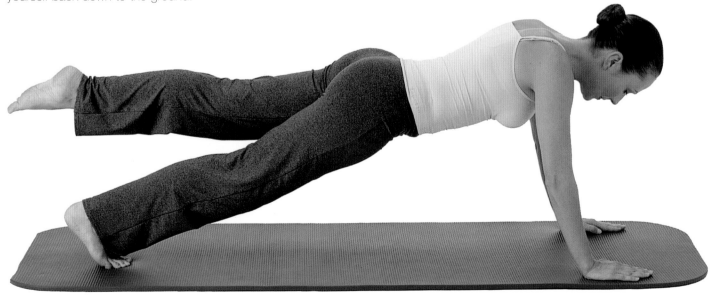

the crab

intermediate/advanced

This is another rolling exercise that requires a great deal of control. It strengthens the core abdominal muscles and also helps to open out the lower back, improving flexibility. It can be tricky to master and you may find that you lose your balance and roll off to one side. Persevere and you will be surprised at how quickly you improve. This exercise is best avoided by anyone with knee or lower-back problems.

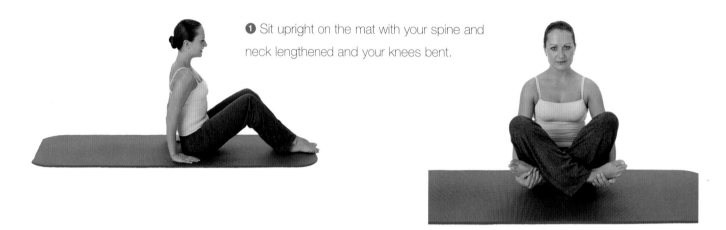

❶ Sit upright on the mat with your spine and neck lengthened and your knees bent.

❷ Raise your feet off the floor, find your point of balance, and cross your ankles, grasping your left foot with your right hand and your right foot with your left hand to hold them in position. Think of pulling your knees in toward your shoulders.

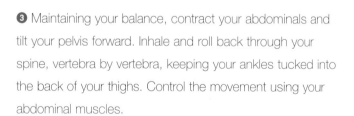

❸ Maintaining your balance, contract your abdominals and tilt your pelvis forward. Inhale and roll back through your spine, vertebra by vertebra, keeping your ankles tucked into the back of your thighs. Control the movement using your abdominal muscles.

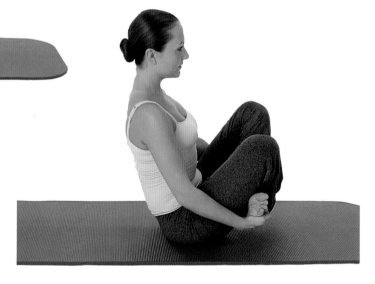

❹ When you reach the furthest point of the roll, exhale and roll slowly back up to a sitting position, keeping your balance, so that your ankles remain crossed and your feet do not need to touch the floor. Repeat the movement five to ten times.

one leg circles (side)

intermediate/advanced

This exercise works the abdominals, stretches and strengthens the buttock and leg muscles, and mobilizes the hip joint. Remember to keep your body in neutral throughout this move, with your spine lengthened and parallel to the floor. Avoid tilting the uppermost hip or shoulder forward as you circle your legs. Do not be concerned if your hips make a slight clicking sound—it is simply an indication of tightness of the ligaments in this area. However, this exercise should be avoided if you feel any pain or discomfort in the hip area or the lower back.

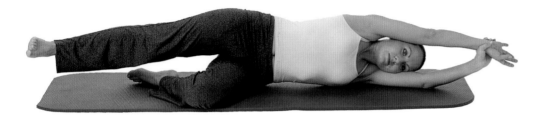

❶ Lie on your left side with your spine in the neutral position, your knees bent up toward your body. Lengthen through your back and neck and take your arms above your head in line with your body, stretching your right arm and clasping your right wrist with your left hand. Support your head on your left arm and look straight ahead. Inhale as you extend your right leg down until it is in line with your body, with your right foot flexed.

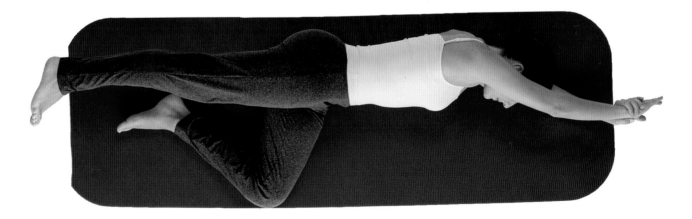

❷ Exhale, contracting your abdominals as you raise your right leg upward to hip level. Still exhaling, draw five to ten small circles with the right foot in a clockwise direction. Pause, inhale, and as you exhale, draw five to ten counterclockwise circles. Keep your knee soft and lengthen your leg away from the hip as you circle—think of the movement as generating from the hip socket itself and not simply the foot. Inhale as you release your right leg back down to the floor. Repeat for your left leg.

the side kick

This exercise allows you to stretch while also working on improving your balance and control. Your body needs to be held in neutral, with your spine lengthened and parallel to the floor. This can be a challenge, as you are positioned on your side and will therefore need to work against gravity. Avoid sinking at your waist—there should be a small gap between your waist and the floor. The forward and back kicks need to be done at a steady, controlled pace.

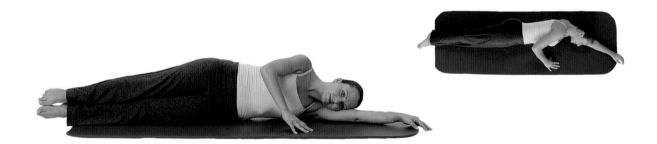

❶ Lie on your side with your body in a straight line, legs together. Your lower arm should lie straight along the floor, with your head resting on it. The other hand rests on the floor in front of your body, to act as a support and help you to keep your balance. Maintain neutral in this position with your shoulders and hips parallel (avoid letting the raised hip drop forward) and your spine lengthened.

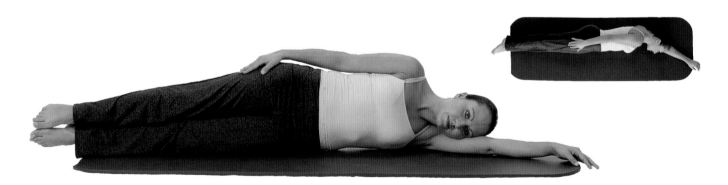

❷ If you are able to balance easily in this position while keeping your body in neutral, you can try resting the top arm along the side of your body instead. If you find you start to wobble, rest the hand back in the original position.

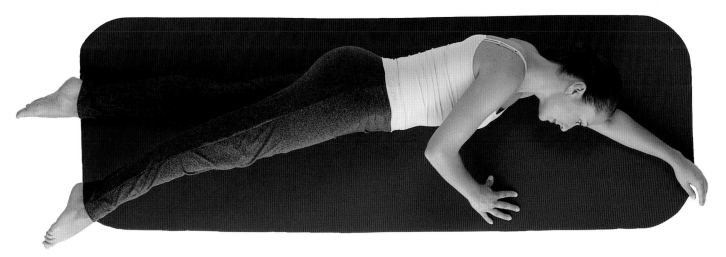

3 If you have not already done so, place the upper hand back onto the floor for support. Inhale, contract your abdominals, and keeping your legs together, raise them slightly from the floor as you exhale. Keeping both legs lifted, inhale and lift the top leg, exhale and take it forward a little, and inhale as you bring it back to center. The movement should be very small to start with, gradually increasing in size with each repetition. It is essential that you keep the alignment of your body throughout this exercise—avoid taking your leg so far forward that it throws you off balance or out of alignment.

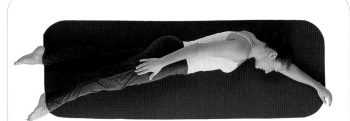

VARIATION: intermediate/advanced

This variation provides you with an extra challenge, as you no longer rely on your hand to help you balance. It is essential that you keep your abdominals contracted and maintain your spine in neutral position, with arms and hips parallel, in order to get the full benefit of this very precise exercise.

Repeat the exercise, but this time without the help of the supporting arm. Gently rest the top arm along the side of your body, keeping it as relaxed as possible.

one leg stretch

beginner

This stretch works to strengthen the abdominal core, improves flexibility in the hip flexors, and is particularly good for anyone with any tightness or stiffness in this area. The basic level provides an excellent stretch for beginners and can be used as a gentle warm-up preparation to the more difficult variations for the more experienced.

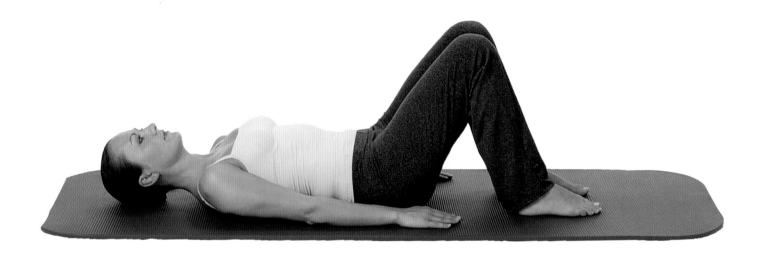

❶ Lie on the floor with your legs bent, knees pointing up to the ceiling, feet parallel, and your arms by your sides with palms facing downward. Your spine should be in neutral with a small gap between your waist and the floor—just enough for you to slide your hand under your lower back. Inhale and contract the abdominal muscles, and as you exhale, extend your left leg, sliding your heel along the ground. Focus on keeping your spine in neutral and your hips level. Inhale as you slide your leg back to the starting position. Repeat on the other side. Alternate your legs for a total of ten to twenty repetitions.

VARIATION 1 beginner/intermediate

When you are confident in your ability to work your legs while keeping your spine in neutral, your hips level, and your abdominals contracted, try this development.

❶ Keeping your spine in neutral, with your hips relaxed and your eyes focused up toward the ceiling, inhale, then as you exhale, contract your abdominals and lift your right leg, with the knee at a right angle, until the shin is parallel to the floor.

❷ Holding your right leg in this position, inhale, then exhale, contract the abdominals, and slide the left leg away from you, keeping the heel in contact with the ground, as in Step 1.

❸ Inhale and return your left leg to the starting position. Repeat this stretch five to ten times, holding the raised leg at right angles and keeping the hips level. Inhale. As you exhale, lower the raised leg. Repeat for the other side.

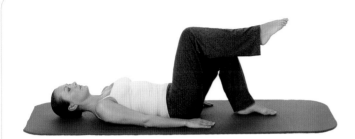
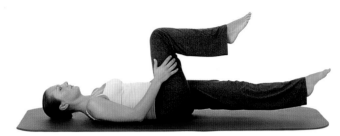

VARIATION 2: intermediate/advanced

This variation is very similar to the procedure described in Variation 1, except that you alternate your legs as you stretch.

❶ Lying on the floor in neutral with knees raised and feet flat on the floor, inhale, then as you exhale, contract your abdominals slightly and lift your right leg until the knee is at a right angle, with the shin parallel to the floor.

❷ Holding your leg in this position and keeping the hips level, inhale, then exhale, contract your abdominals, and slide your left leg away from you, keeping the heel in contact with the ground. Inhale and return your left leg to the starting position, continuing through this position to allow it to float up to join your right leg (knee bent, shin parallel to the floor).

❸ Exhale as you now lower your right leg, again continuing the movement through this position and sliding your heel along the ground to extend your leg out in front of you. Inhale as you slide your right leg back to the starting position, floating it up to meet your left leg. Repeat this stretch ten to twenty times, holding the raised leg at a right angle and keeping the hips level.

VARIATION 3: advanced

Once you have developed sufficient strength and flexibility, you are ready for this challenging variation. If you suffer any discomfort with this version or find yourself unable to isolate your legs while keeping your body in alignment with the hips level, you need to return to a less challenging level for a while.

❶ Follow the instructions for Step 1, in Variation 2, then, holding your right leg in this position, inhale, then exhale and slide your left leg away from you. Inhale and raise your left leg, bending at the knee and floating it up to the right-angle position with the shin parallel to the floor. At the same time, do the reverse with your right leg, lowering and extending it out in front of you. Keep this lowered leg a few inches above the ground as you extend it. If this is too difficult, raise the position of the extended leg so that it is at more of an angle to the floor. This will be less demanding on the abdominal muscles. The feet should be relaxed and in a soft point.

❷ Exhale and lower your left leg as you raise the right. Repeat a total of ten to twenty times, making sure that the movement is rhythmic and controlled, in time with your breathing. Use your hands to guide you and help improve coordination by gently grasping each thigh in turn with both hands as you raise it toward your face.

double arm stretch 1

beginner

This stretch works at strengthening the abdominal muscles, while challenging you to sustain the neutral position of your spine throughout the movement.

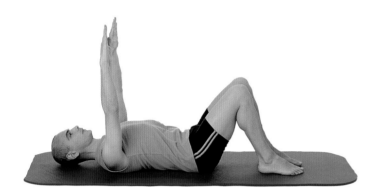

❶ Lie on the floor with your spine in neutral, legs bent, knees and ankles hip-width apart, arms by your sides, feet flat on the floor. Relax your shoulders, drawing the shoulder blades back and down behind you. Inhale, then exhale, contracting your abdominals. Keeping your spine in neutral, inhale and bring your arms up to shoulder level, hands shoulder-width apart, pointing straight up to the ceiling.

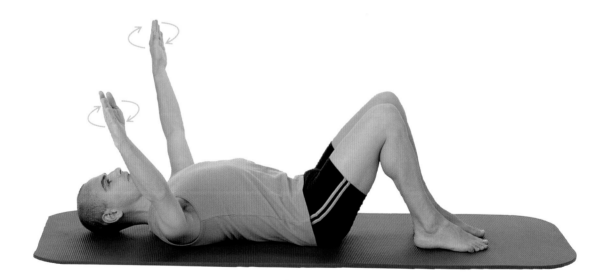

❷ Now take your arms out into a circular motion, making small circles with your arms, hands moving in opposite directions. Exhale as you take your arms out away from your body and inhale as you bring them back in again. Repeat five times. Make sure your arms and shoulders stay relaxed throughout, with your shoulder blades drawn down and back behind you. The movement should be as smooth and flowing as possible.

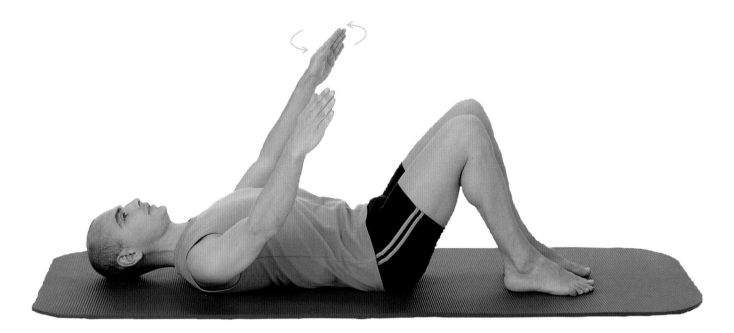

❸ Change the direction of your arms, exhaling as you take your hands down toward your body, then inhaling as you bring them up and around. Repeat five times. Change direction again and repeat the sequence one more time, making five circles in one direction, then five circles in the other. Gradually make the circles bigger, but make sure that you are able to maintain your spine in the neutral position with abdominals contracted. If you find that you are experiencing any tension or soreness in your shoulders, you can slide your arms along the floor in the downward stage of the circles.

VARIATION: beginner/intermediate

Once you have mastered the above sequence, keeping your spine in neutral as you perform your arm circles, you are ready to increase the difficulty and make the abdominal muscles work a little harder still. Avoid dropping the lowered leg out to the side; keep it in the parallel position with the knee pointing straight up to the ceiling.

Follow the instructions for the above sequence, but this time, once you have raised your arms to shoulder height, allow your right leg to float upward until the shin is parallel to the floor, keeping the knee at a ninety-degree angle. Holding your leg in this position, continue the exercise. Do five circles in each

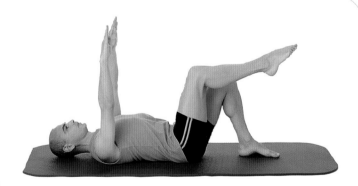

direction, then pause and switch legs, floating your right leg back down to the floor and then your left leg up to the right-angle position. Do five circles in each direction in this position, then bring your leg back down and lower your arms.

shoulder bridge

beginner/intermediate/advanced

This is an excellent exercise for increasing the mobility in your spine and improving the strength and muscle control in your abdominal and pelvic areas.

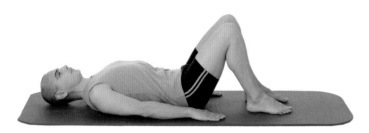

❶ Lie on the floor with your legs hip-width apart, knees bent, feet flat on the floor, heels approximately under your knees (or as close as is comfortable), and arms resting by your sides. Lengthen through your spine and along the back of your neck.

❷ Inhale and then exhale, contracting your abdominals and tilting the pelvis upward very slightly, lifting the tailbone off the floor. Inhale and release back down to the floor. Repeat, lifting a little more of the tailbone off the mat each time. Think of peeling your spine off the floor, vertebra by vertebra, exhaling as you lift and inhaling as you release your spine back down to the floor, using a smooth, controlled motion. Keep the hips level and the knees stable as you carry out this sequence. Repeat three to five times.

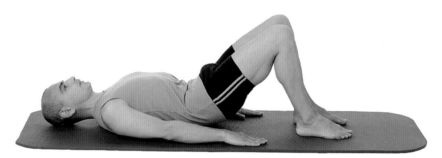

❸ Inhale and then exhale, contracting your abdominals and rolling the tailbone up off the floor onto your shoulders, until your body reaches a diagonal line (like a ski slope), with your spine in neutral. Inhale and then exhale as you contract your abdominals and roll your spine slowly back down to the starting position. Repeat three to five times.

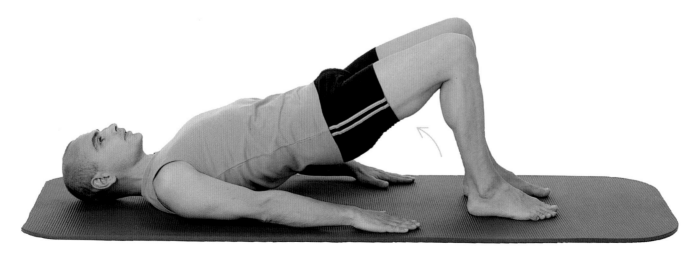

VARIATION 1: intermediate

Once you have built up sufficient strength in your abdominals and are able to keep the alignment of your body as you roll up and down through your spine, you are ready to add this variation to the sequence.

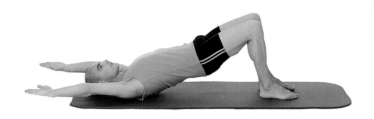

Follow the instructions for Step 3, but this time, once you reach the ski slope position, inhale and raise your arms up over your head and then back to the starting position. Exhale as you roll your spine back down to the floor. To increase the challenge, keep your arms over your head while you exhale and roll back down, then inhale as you bring your arms back. Repeat five to ten times.

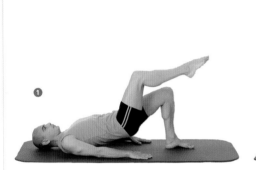
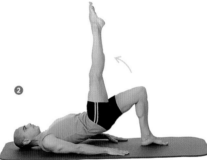
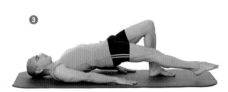

VARIATION 2: advanced

The challenge with this development is to maintain the alignment and stability of your body as you raise one leg off the floor. Build up this sequence slowly, one step at a time, only adding the next development once you have gained confidence with the previous one.

❶ Follow the instructions for Step 3, but this time holding the ski slope position. Now inhale and float your right leg up off the ground in a bent position.

❷ Exhale and continue extending your leg until it is pointing straight up toward the ceiling. Use the contraction in your abdominals to help you remain stable. Check that your spine is in neutral with the hips level. Inhale.

❸ Exhale and lower the extended leg straight down until it is parallel with the floor, keeping your hips level and lifted off the ground. Inhale and then exhale, contract your abdominals, and raise your extended leg back up until your toes are pointing up toward the ceiling once more. Inhale as you bend your right knee and float your leg back down to the ski slope position. Exhale as you roll down through your spine to return to the starting position.

side bend prep

beginner/intermediate

The Side Bend Prep is a strength-building exercise that also works to improve your muscle control as you focus on lifting your hips while maintaining your body in its correct alignment.

❶ Sit on your left side, knees bent, legs parallel, knees, ankles, and feet together, hips stacked one on top of the other. Place your left arm on the floor to support you, elbow directly under the shoulder, forearm resting on the floor with your hand pointing straight out in front of you, upper arm in line with your left shoulder. Rest your right arm on the floor in front of you. Your eyes should focus straight in front of you throughout this sequence. Lengthen through your spine, lifting your ribs so that your body is straight, creating a right-angle triangle between your body, your lowered arm, and the floor.

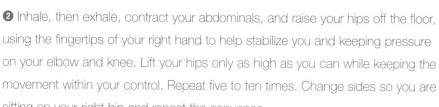

❷ Inhale, then exhale, contract your abdominals, and raise your hips off the floor, using the fingertips of your right hand to help stabilize you and keeping pressure on your elbow and knee. Lift your hips only as high as you can while keeping the movement within your control. Repeat five to ten times. Change sides so you are sitting on your right hip and repeat the sequence.

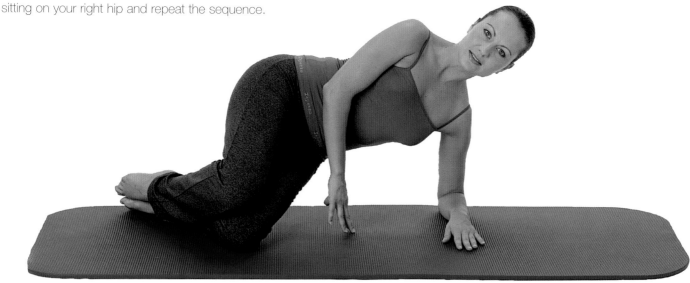

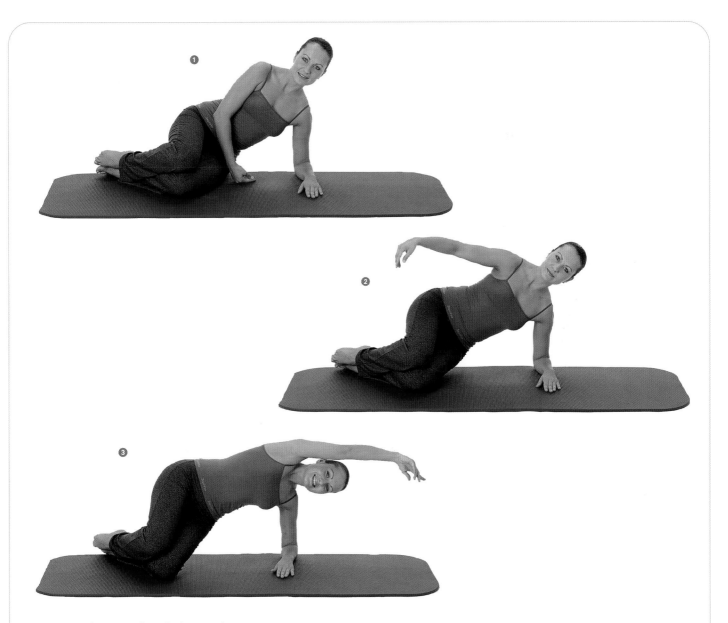

VARIATION: intermediate/advanced

Try to keep your body in a line throughout this variation—avoid the uppermost shoulder and hip rounding forward as you lift up and stretch your arm over your head.

❶ Begin the sequence as described in Step 1. Your right arm rests in front of your body with the palm facing up.

❷ Inhale, then exhale, contracting your abdominals and raising your hips off the floor, keeping pressure on your elbow and knee. As you lift your hips, float your right arm upward, making sure it is in line with your body, elbow curved slightly forward.

❸ Holding your body in position, keep curving your arm over the head in a smooth, controlled movement, as if you are drawing a semicircle in the air. As you extend your arm, creating a stretch along the right side of your body, avoid dropping your hips or tipping them forward. Keep lengthening up through your spine and along the back of your neck. When you have extended as far as you can (maintaining control and keeping your body aligned), inhale, float your arm back along the same semicircular path, and then lower your hips. Repeat five to ten times. Change sides and repeat the sequence.

side kick (kneeling)

intermediate/advanced

This exercise improves balance and coordination, and also works the waistline, hips, and legs. Try to keep your body stationary as you carry out the kicking movement with your legs. Avoid this movement if you suffer from any knee problems.

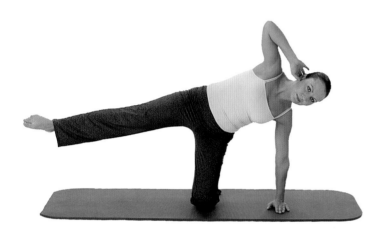

❶ Kneel on the floor with your legs placed slightly apart. Lengthen up through your spine and the back of your neck. Position your left hand directly below your left shoulder, fingertips pointing forward. Raise your right arm, placing your fingertips lightly at the back of your head. Extend your right leg out along the floor in line with your body, pointing your toe. Keep your shoulders dropped away from your ears, pulling down and back with your shoulder blades. Inhale, then exhale, contracting your abdominals and allowing your right leg to float upward toward the ceiling, keeping it extended and bringing it up to hip height, making sure it is still in line with your body.

❷ Inhale, and as you exhale, take your leg forward a few inches, keeping it at hip height, then inhale once more as you bring your leg back. Avoid tilting your uppermost hip forward and make sure you maintain the abdominal contraction throughout the exercise. Repeat five to ten times without lowering your leg. Repeat the same sequence for the other side of your body.

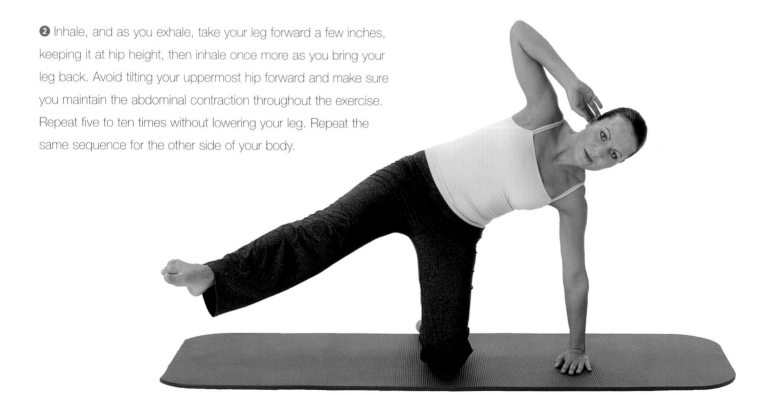

side bend stretch

beginner/intermediate

This exercise creates a stretch along your waist, up the side of your body, and along your arm, while also creating a stretch to the muscles of the extended leg. As your flexibility increases, you will be able to intensify the stretch by curving your body further over the extended leg toward the knee. Keep lengthening up through your spine and along the back of your neck throughout the movement.

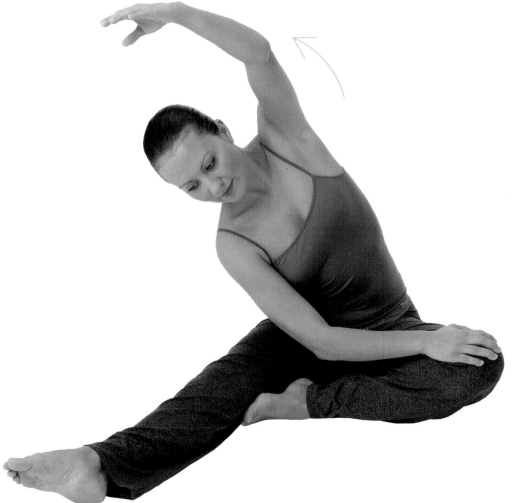

❶ Sit in an upright position with your legs apart, knees soft, and arms stretched out to the sides at just below shoulder height. Bend your left knee and draw the left foot in to rest against the inner thigh of your right leg. Inhale, contract your abdominals, and exhale, curving your torso over toward your right knee, taking your left arm up and over your head, and at the same time allowing your right hand to float down and rest lightly on your left knee. Keep stretching as you exhale, imagining that you are lifting your body up out of your waist and over a beach ball, to avoid collapsing the ribs on the right side of your body and also to increase the stretch on your left side. Inhale and come back to center, then exhale as you curve over to the right once again. Repeat the stretch five to ten times to the right, trying to increase the stretch with each repetition. Switch your leg positions and repeat the sequence for the other side.

scissors

beginner/intermediate/advanced

This is a challenging move, even at beginner level, and it requires a great deal of concentration in order to coordinate your breathing with the movement of your limbs. It works to improve the strength and flexibility of your legs and hip flexors. Although this appears to be a leg movement, the movements actually generate from the abdominal muscles.

❶ Lie on the floor with your legs bent, knees pointing up to the ceiling, feet parallel, and your arms by your sides. Make sure that your spine is in neutral and your neck and shoulders are relaxed.

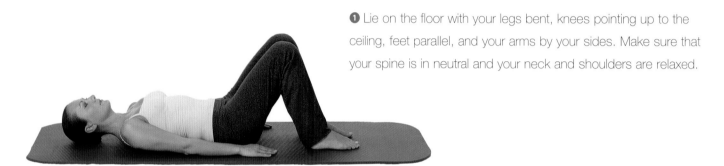

❷ Keeping your hips level and your eyes focused up toward the ceiling, inhale, then as you exhale, contract your abdominals slightly and lift your right leg until your shin is parallel to the floor with your knee at a right angle.

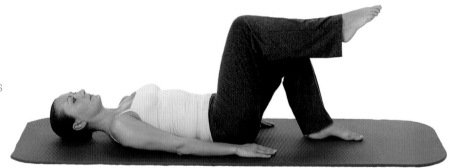

❸ Making sure the bend of your knee stays at a right angle, inhale, then exhale and dip the toes of your right foot down toward the floor, as if into an imaginary pool of water. Repeat five times and then return your leg to the starting position. Repeat for your other leg. If you are unable to dip the foot all the way down to the floor and keep your spine in neutral and your hips level, then just dip the foot as far as you can. Over time you will gradually build up strength and will be able to take the movement further.

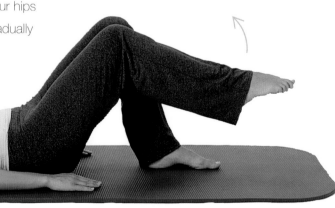

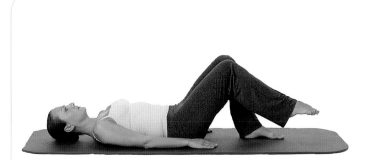

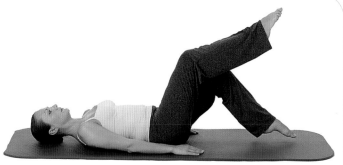

VARIATION 1: intermediate

Follow the instructions for Step 3, but this time increase the angle of the knee bend so that your leg is extended out slightly and lowered a little more toward the floor, intensifying the effect on the abdominal muscles. This variation is more challenging than you might expect, so concentrate on contracting your abdominal muscles and keeping your spine in the neutral position and your hips level. Check that your neck is lengthened and your eyes focused straight above you. Repeat five to ten times on each leg.

VARIATION 2: intermediate/advanced

Follow the instructions for Step 3, this time extending the angle of your leg further to increase the intensity of the movement and alternating your legs each time. As one leg returns to the starting position, the other leg rises off the floor. Alternate your breathing as you raise and lower your legs. Do the movement at an even pace, ensuring your legs are both raised and lowered at a controlled, even rhythm in time with your breathing. Repeat five to ten times on each leg.

VARIATION 3: advanced

For the advanced version of this exercise, begin by lying on the floor in neutral (as in Step 1), then lengthen your legs, one at a time, along the ground. Inhale and contract your abdominals, then exhale as you raise your right leg, keeping it straight, but with soft knees. Inhale and lower your right leg as you raise your left, then exhale as you lower your left leg and raise your right. Keep your legs in a parallel position throughout the movement; keep them from opening out to the side as this will change the position of your pelvis. Your legs should work in isolation, with your hips remaining level and your abdominals contracted. Depending on the strength of your abdominal muscles, you can either do this movement with your legs held quite high, or to increase the challenge, lowering your legs

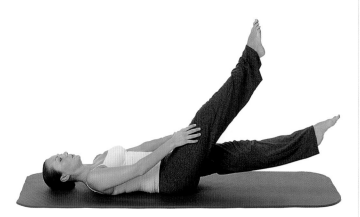

down toward the floor as you make the scissoring action. To help improve coordination and engage the upper body, you can add your hands into the exercise, gently grasping alternate legs as they are raised. Repeat the scissoring action ten to twenty times.

one leg circles

beginner

The focus of this exercise is to work your abdominals and leg muscles, while at the same time maintaining the alignment of your body and developing core abdominal and pelvic strength. Your leg circles should be small, subtle movements, which serve to improve the flexibility and strength of your leg muscles and hip joints. You may find that your hips make a clicking sound when you start this exercise. This is not a problem, unless it is painful. It is simply an indication of the tightness of the ligaments in this area.

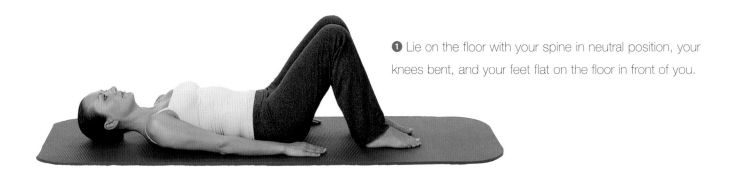

❶ Lie on the floor with your spine in neutral position, your knees bent, and your feet flat on the floor in front of you.

❷ Keeping your spine in neutral, with your hips relaxed and your eyes focused up toward the ceiling, inhale, then as you exhale, contract your abdominals slightly and lift your right leg until your shin is parallel to the floor, with your knee roughly at a right angle. Place the fingertips of your right hand on your right knee. Inhale, and as you exhale, draw five to ten small circles with your knee in a clockwise direction, using your fingertips to guide you. Pause, inhale, and as you exhale, draw five to ten small circles, this time in a counterclockwise direction. Think of the circling movement as generating from your hip socket and imagine your hip releasing as you progress through this exercise. Make sure you keep your opposite leg still, with your knee pointing straight up toward the ceiling. Inhale, releasing your right leg back down to the floor as you exhale, and dropping your hand to your side. Repeat with your left leg.

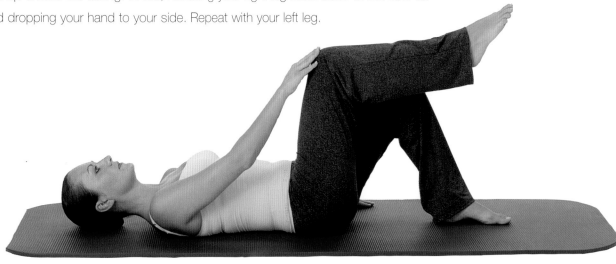

VARIATION 1: intermediate

Once you have mastered this exercise and are able to make controlled, even circles with your knee, you no longer need your hand to guide you and can let it rest at the side of your body. Gradually increase the size of the circles, remembering to maintain a slow, flowing movement and making sure it is in time with the breathing. Do five to ten circles, first clockwise, then counterclockwise, on each leg.

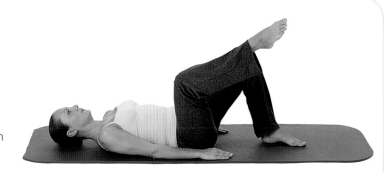

VARIATION 2: advanced

When you feel ready for a further challenge, straighten the raised leg toward the ceiling and draw circles with your feet. Keep your knee soft and think of lengthening your leg out away from the hip. Do ten circles, first clockwise, then counterclockwise, on each leg. Only attempt this variation once you are confident with the previous levels of this movement. It can be very challenging to maintain your core stability and neutral spine if you are not yet sufficiently strong and flexible in the lower back and abdominals and pelvic area. If you experience any tension in your neck or lower back, or have difficulty in keeping your hips level and your abdominals contracted, then you need to return to one of the previous versions of this movement.

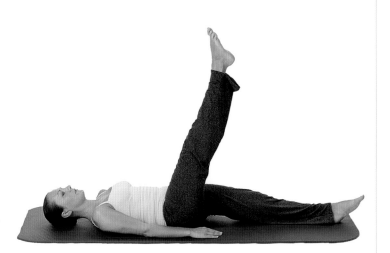

jackknife

intermediate/advanced

You will need to have developed a certain amount of strength in your abdominals and flexibility in your spine before attempting this exercise. To maximize its effect as a strength-building move, it needs to be carried out as slowly as possible. Remember to use your abdominal muscles to control your body as you roll through your spine.

❶ Lie on your back with your legs extended, feet pointed, knees and ankles together. Let your arms rest by your sides, palms facing downward. Pull the shoulder blades down and back, making sure your spine is in neutral, with the back of your neck lengthened. Focus the eyes straight up at the ceiling.

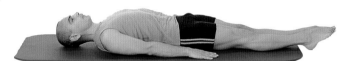

❷ Inhale, then exhale, contract your abdominals, tilt the pelvis forward, squeeze the inner thighs together, squeeze your buttocks, and lift your legs to form a ninety-degree angle to your body. Continuing the movement, peel your tailbone and lower spine away from the floor. If necessary, use your arms to support you, pressing down on the floor with the hands to stabilize yourself. Inhale, then exhale, contracting your abdominals, slowly roll back down through your spine, vertebra by vertebra, and lower your legs. Repeat ten times.

VARIATION: advanced

This challenging version of the Jackknife builds strength in your abdominal core and arms, while stretching the muscles of your back, shoulders, and neck. As you roll up, avoid rolling onto your neck—keep the weight of your body on your shoulders. Keep lengthening your legs and squeezing the inner thighs together throughout.

Follow the instructions given above, this time continuing to peel your spine off the floor as you exhale, until you are resting on your shoulders, neck, and arms, with your body and legs in a straight line pointing up toward the ceiling. Again, use your arms and hands to help balance you, but try to control the entire movement with your abdominal core. Inhale and roll back down to the starting position, using a slow, even, controlled movement, keeping your feet positioned directly above your face for as long as possible. Repeat ten times.

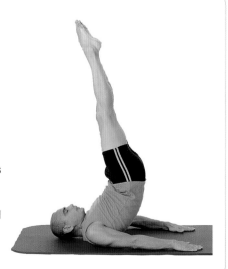

hip twist

intermediate/advanced

This exercise improves strength in the abdominal core. Aim to keep your torso perfectly still as you rotate your legs. Keep lengthening up through your spine and the back of your neck throughout the exercise, and allow your arm position to create a slight stretch across your shoulders and chest.

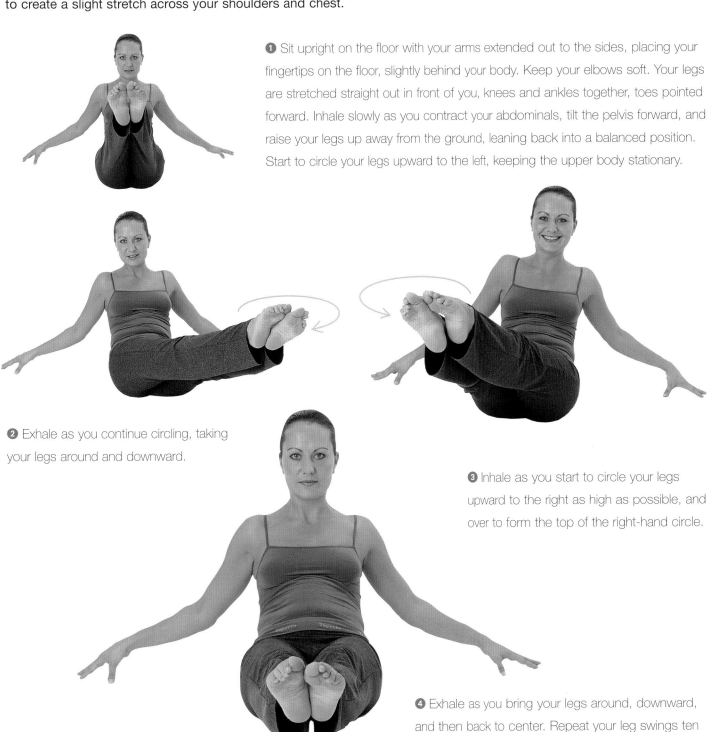

❶ Sit upright on the floor with your arms extended out to the sides, placing your fingertips on the floor, slightly behind your body. Keep your elbows soft. Your legs are stretched straight out in front of you, knees and ankles together, toes pointed forward. Inhale slowly as you contract your abdominals, tilt the pelvis forward, and raise your legs up away from the ground, leaning back into a balanced position. Start to circle your legs upward to the left, keeping the upper body stationary.

❷ Exhale as you continue circling, taking your legs around and downward.

❸ Inhale as you start to circle your legs upward to the right as high as possible, and over to form the top of the right-hand circle.

❹ Exhale as you bring your legs around, downward, and then back to center. Repeat your leg swings ten times for each direction.

one leg kick

intermediate/advanced

This stretches the thigh muscles and your abdominals, and strengthens the hamstrings, the hip flexors, the muscles of the chest area, and the arms. The technique for this move requires strength, balance, good muscle control, and stability. If you suffer from knee problems, it is best to either leave this exercise out of your program entirely or to follow the instructions for the variation given below, slowly stretching your heel toward your buttock, instead of using a kicking motion.

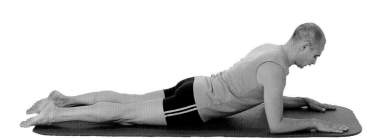

❶ Lie face down, with your legs parallel and placed slightly apart, soles of the feet facing upward. Your arms are positioned close to your body, forearms in contact with the floor, palms placed on the floor on either side of your shoulders, elbows soft. Stretching through your chest, raise your shoulders off the ground. Adjust your hand position so that your elbows are positioned directly below your shoulders, hands stretching forward. Lengthen through your spine and along the back of your neck, eyes focused down between your hands.

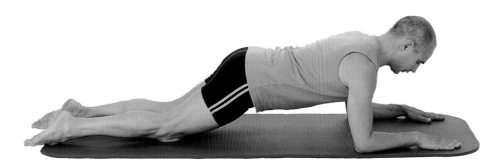

❷ Inhale and then exhale, contracting your abdominal muscles and lifting your hips away from the floor, bringing the weight onto your knees. Inhale and contract your abdominals, lengthening out through your spine and the back of your neck.

❸ Keeping the contraction in your abdominals, continue to exhale as you raise your right leg, extending and lengthening it, toes pointed away from your body. Keep your hips level and avoid lifting the extended leg too high—try to keep it at the same height as the rest of your body.

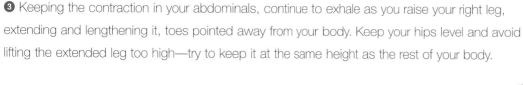

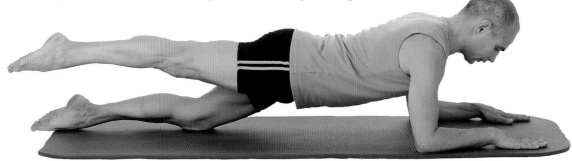

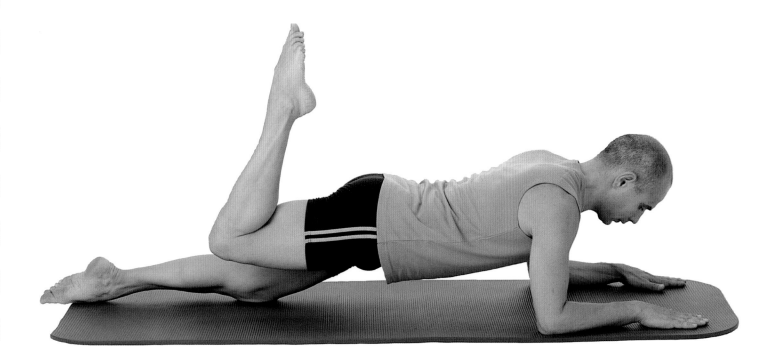

❹ Inhale and snap-kick your right heel toward your right buttock. Exhale and extend your right leg back down to the floor, transfer the weight onto your right knee, and extend your left leg. Inhale and snap-kick your left heel toward your left buttock. Exhale and release your left leg back down to the floor. Repeat the exercise ten times on each side.

VARIATION: intermediate

If you have any difficulty in keeping your body balanced and aligned while doing the above sequence, or if you experience any discomfort in your shoulders or knees, then try the following variation:

❶ Position yourself as described in Step 1. Then, if you are finding it too much of a struggle to lift your chest and straighten your arms, keep your forearms in contact with the floor and simply stretch through your chest to raise your upper body a little.

❷ Lengthen through your spine and along the back of your neck, eyes focused down and forward between your hands. Keeping your hips pressed evenly into the floor, inhale and bend your right knee, curving the right foot up toward the ceiling (keeping the thigh in contact with the floor). Exhale and kick your heel toward your buttock, then release your leg back so that it is pointing up to the ceiling, then kick again. Inhale and release your right leg back down to the ground and raise your left leg. Repeat the kicking sequence for your left leg. Repeat five times on each leg, keeping the contraction in your abdominals.

teaser

intermediate/advanced

The aim of this strength-building exercise is to raise and lower your body to a balanced position without relying on your legs or arms to help you, while keeping your lower body perfectly still. Keep your shoulders down, with your shoulder blades pulled down and back throughout this entire sequence, and make sure the movement is smooth and controlled at all times.

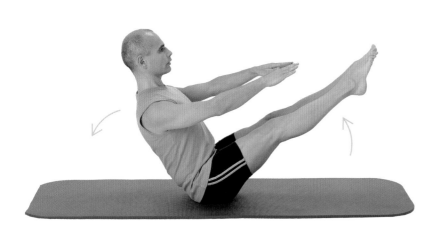

❶ Sit on the floor with your legs straight out in front of you, knees and ankles together, toes softly pointed, hands placed palms-down beside your hips, fingers pointing straight forward. Lengthen up through your spine and the back of your neck. Inhale, exhale, contract your abdominals, and lift your legs up off the floor, squeezing your inner thighs together and leaning back until you find your position of balance. Inhale slowly, raising your arms until they are parallel with your leg position.

❷ Continue the movement, rolling your back down onto the mat, one vertebra at a time, as far as you can, using your abdominal muscles to control the movement and keeping your legs in the raised position. Inhale, then exhale and roll back up to sitting. Repeat five to ten times without lowering your legs. To finish, inhale as you lower your arms back to your sides, then exhale as you slowly lower your legs down to the floor.

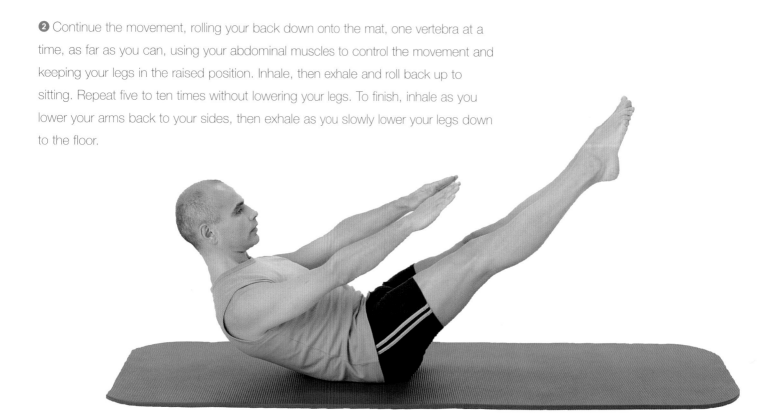

VARIATION 1: intermediate/advanced

This variation is a little easier, as you keep one foot on the ground for stability, but it has the added challenge of twisting your upper body to one side and then the other, stretching and strengthening the mid-back and obliques. Keep the abdominal contraction as you twist.

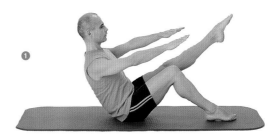

❶ Follow the instructions for Steps 1 and 2, but start with your feet flat on the floor, knees bent. Raise only your left foot off the ground, extending your leg so that your thighs remain parallel and leaving your right foot on the floor. Roll down your spine onto the mat as far as you can, again using your abdominal muscles to control the movement and keeping your left leg in the raised position. Inhale, then exhale and roll back up to sitting. Continuing the movement, rotate at your waist, twisting slightly to the right, and lengthen through your spine to stretch forward over your right knee. Make sure that you generate this movement from the stretch through your spine, and not by just

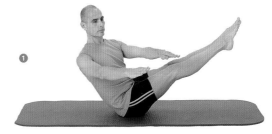

reaching forward with your arms. Inhale as you come back to center and then roll back down to the floor.

❷ Repeat the stretch, rotating your torso to the left. Repeat the sequence five to ten times.

VARIATION 2: advanced

This works to increase the strength in the central core, while improving balance and coordination. Keep lengthening up through your spine and neck throughout the exercise. If you feel discomfort in the lower back, stop and return to previous levels.

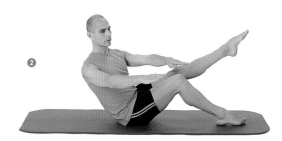

❶ Start with your legs straight out in front of you, knees and ankles together, toes pointed, hands placed palms-down beside the hips, fingers pointing straight forward. Lengthen up through your spine and the back of your neck. Inhale, exhale, contract your abdominals, and lift your legs up off the floor, squeezing the inner thighs together, and leaning back into a balanced position. Inhale slowly, raising your arms until they are parallel with your leg position. Exhale and roll back as far as you can, keeping your legs raised as in the original version described above. Inhale, then exhale as you roll back up to sitting. Rotate at the waist, twisting to the right, and stretch

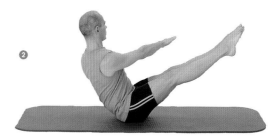

forward, lengthening your spine, over your right knee. Inhale, come back to center, and roll back down onto the floor.

❷ Repeat the stretch, rotating your torso to the left. Repeat the sequence five to ten times.

neck pull prep

intermediate/advanced

This movement is a preparation exercise for Neck Pull Prone and requires strength and mobility in your abdominals and lower back. The exercise works your abdominal muscles and helps to increase the flexibility of your spine. Remember, it is essential to maintain the correct body position, with your abdominals contracted and your pelvis tucked under, through all these variations. This will help you to avoid any stress or strain to your lower back. However, if you feel any discomfort, stop—chances are that you are not yet quite ready for this demanding move.

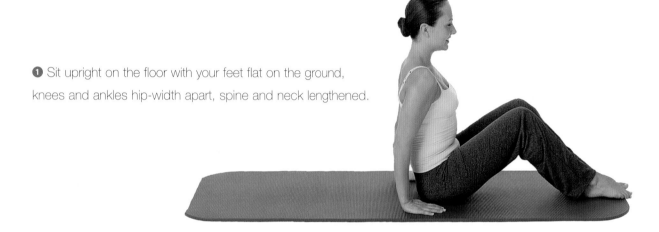

❶ Sit upright on the floor with your feet flat on the ground, knees and ankles hip-width apart, spine and neck lengthened.

❷ Inhale, contract your abdominals, exhale, and tilt your pelvis forward, allowing yourself to curl back slightly, vertebra by vertebra. Keep your eyes focused forward, chin tucked in slightly to create a gentle stretch through the back of your neck. When you reach the point where you start to feel resistance in your abdominal muscles, hold the position and allow your left arm to float straight up until it is positioned just in front of your ears, keeping your shoulders down and away from your ears and your elbow soft. Inhale, releasing your arm back down to your side and rolling slowly back up to the sitting position. Do the same movement, this time raising your right arm. Repeat three to five times on each side.

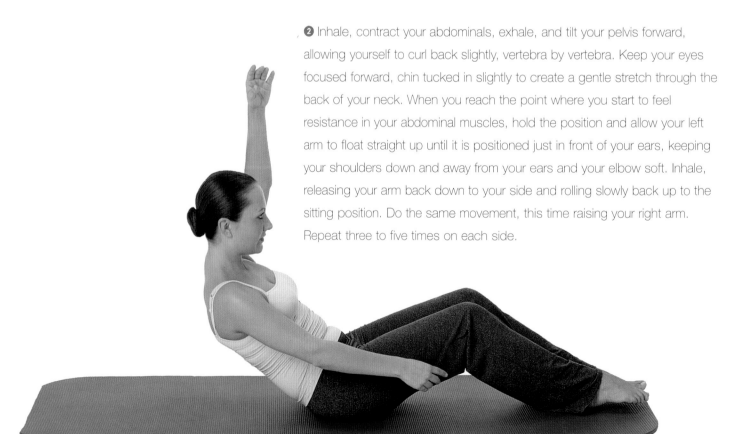

VARIATION 1: advanced

Once you have mastered the above exercise, you are ready to progress to this variation. This version is the same as that given above, but using both arms together. You will need to work harder at keeping your shoulders down and your neck lengthened. Remember to use the pelvic tilt to initiate the curling-down movement.

❶ Sit upright on the floor with your feet flat on the ground, knees and ankles hip-width apart, spine and neck lengthened.

❷ Follow the procedure for Step 2, this time allowing both arms to float up to the side of your head. As you repeat the exercise, try to curl down a little further each time. Repeat the sequence five to ten times. If your abdominal muscles or shoulders start to shake or feel uncomfortable, then return to center and stop the exercise—you have done enough.

VARIATION 2: advanced

❶ If you would like even more of a challenge, then repeat the exercise, this time with either your fingertips resting on your temples, or your hands behind your head, keeping your elbows pointing out to the sides and your shoulder blades drawn down and back. Your chin is tilted slightly down and your neck lengthened into a gentle stretch, but there should be no feeling of tension in your neck as you do this movement.

❷ As you gradually build up strength and flexibility, you will be able to curl back all the way to the floor. Once you have reached the floor, inhale, exhale, contract your abdominals, and roll back up to center, remembering to keep your chin tucked in very slightly and your neck lengthened.

❸ To keep increasing the difficulty, gradually move your feet further away from your body. Eventually you will be able to do the sequence with straight legs. This variation should be done keeping your knees and ankles together, to give yourself more stability.

TIP: Do not attempt any of the more difficult variations until you are confident that you are strong and flexible enough to do so. If you find yourself struggling, return to one of the less challenging levels until you have improved your strength and flexibility.

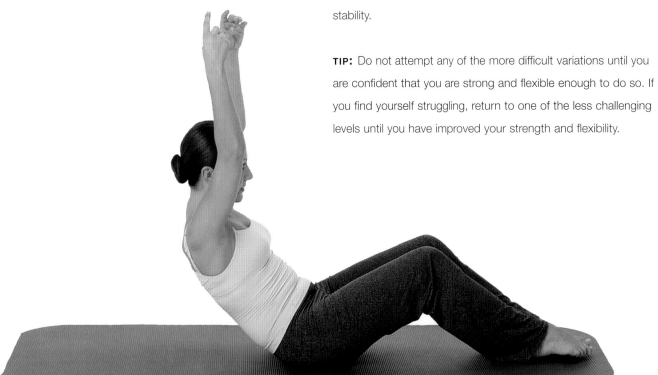

neck pull prone

advanced

This challenging move should only be attempted once you are very familiar with the Pilates technique and have sufficient strength and mobility in your abdominals and lower back. This move is contraindicated for anyone who has sustained a neck injury or suffers from neck problems in any way. Check with your medical practitioner if you are at all concerned.

❶ Lie flat on your back with your spine in neutral and your legs extended, knees and ankles together, your hands behind your head (or with your fingertips at your temples), and your elbows bent. Breathe, allowing your shoulders to relax—imagine them sinking into the floor.

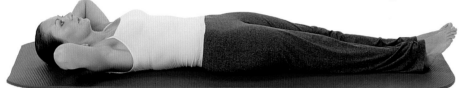

❷ Inhale, then exhale as you contract your abdominals and slowly raise your head, keeping your neck lengthened and your chin very slightly dropped in toward your chest. Curl your spine up off the floor, vertebra by vertebra, raising yourself off the ground a little and keeping your shoulders down. Your hands should rest behind your head, with your arms relaxed, elbows pointing to the sides. When you reach a point where you begin to feel resistance in your abdominal muscles, inhale, then exhale as you contract your abdominals a little further, tilt your pelvis forward, and roll back down to the floor in a slow, graceful movement. Repeat five to ten times.

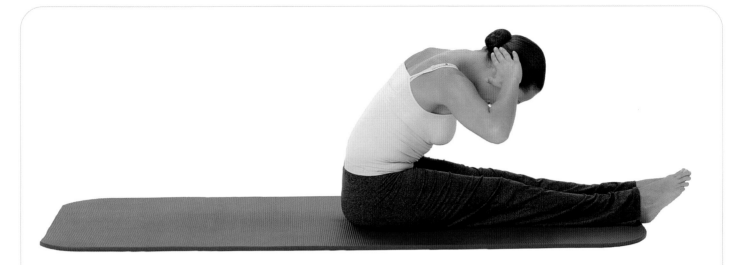

VARIATION: advanced

This move requires additional strength and stability for you to work your abdominals sufficiently deeply to bring yourself up to a sitting position. Keep the movement smooth, avoiding any jerks. If you start to feel any stress in your lower back or find you cannot use your abdominal muscles to continue the movement, then inhale and return to the starting position.

Follow the procedure described above, but this time continue rolling up through your spine until you have reached an upright sitting position. Without stopping the flow of the movement, inhale, then exhale, keeping the abdominal contraction, and curl forward.

the cat

beginner/intermediate

This gentle stretch is particularly effective for relieving tension or stiffness in your back and shoulders, and is an excellent exercise for anyone suffering from tightness or discomfort in the lower back. If your knees feel uncomfortable in this position, place a small folded towel or blanket under your knees to provide extra padding.

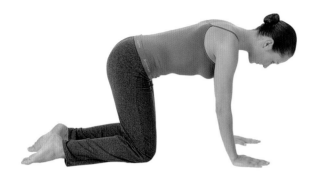

❶ Kneel in the box position—on all fours with your knees hip-width apart, directly below your hips, and your hands directly below your shoulders, fingers pointing forward, away from your body. Keep your arms straight, but avoid locking your elbows. Let your feet rest on the floor, parallel, in a relaxed state, toes pointing away from your body. Focus your eyes down to the floor and lengthen along your spine and back of your neck. Inhale.

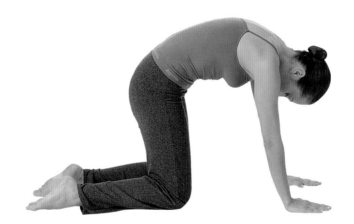

❷ Exhale and contract your abdominals, tuck your pelvis under, drop your chin to your chest, keeping as much length as you can in the back of your neck, and allow your upper back to lift toward the ceiling, creating an arch shape in your upper back. Keep your hips and shoulders level and your knees at a right angle.

❸ Inhale as you release back to center and then reverse the curve, lifting your tailbone to the ceiling, dropping your waist toward the floor and lifting your head, lengthening your neck upward toward the ceiling and away from your spine. Avoid overarching your spine in this position, as this will create pressure in your lower back. Repeat the sequence five to ten times, exhaling as you lift upward, and inhaling as you curve your spine down. The movement should be slow, controlled, and flowing, in time with your breathing.

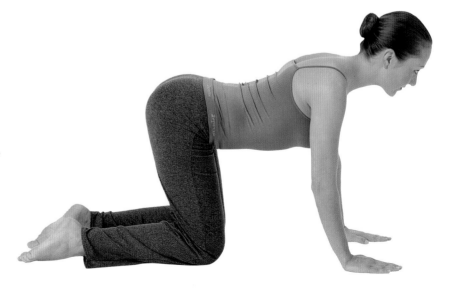

prayer

beginner/intermediate

The Prayer position is a wonderful relaxation pose that allows gravity to work to give a gentle stretch and release to the whole of your spine. Avoid this exercise if you suffer from any knee problems.

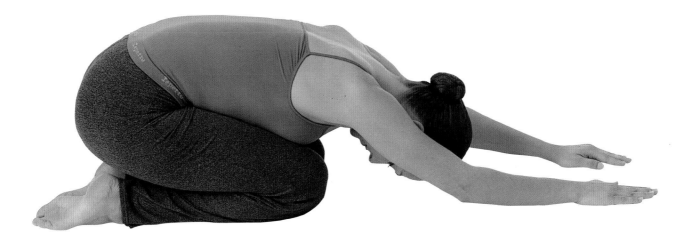

❶ Kneel on all fours, with your knees directly below your hips and your hands directly below your shoulders, fingers pointing forward, away from your body. Lengthen along your spine and back of your neck. Inhale and then exhale, contracting your abdominals and slowly bringing your body back until you are sitting on your heels with your chest resting on your thighs. Leave your arms stretched out in front of you and relax your forehead down to the floor. Avoid hunching your shoulders— keep them dropped with as much space as possible between

your shoulders and the ears. Hold the position for about a minute, longer if you wish, allowing your body to relax a little more with each exhalation. Don't worry if you are unable to sit right back on your heels to start with, just allow your body to relax down as far as it is able to comfortably. Over time, as you gain flexibility in your spine and hips, you will find that this will gradually change, and you will effortlessly be able to reach the tailbone closer to the feet.

VARIATION: beginner/intermediate

This variation is identical to the previous version, except for your arm position. Experiment with the two positions and see which one you prefer. If you have any tension in your neck and shoulders, you may find that this position is the more comfortable one for you, as it gives a slightly different stretch to the shoulder and neck area.

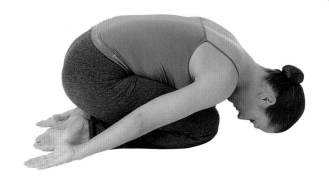

Follow the instructions given for the previous version. As you sit back on your heels, slide your arms back along the floor, close to your sides, with the palms facing upward. Take the

hands back as far as you can and relax your arms and shoulders as you bring your forehead down to the floor. Hold this position for about a minute.

push-up 2

Once you are confident that you have built up sufficient strength with the basic Push-Up, you can move on to this variation. Your aim here is to keep your legs straight throughout the movement, but without straining. If necessary, do the exercise with legs slightly bent until you are used to the movement. If you feel any discomfort in the lower back or the top of your shoulders, return to the previous version of the exercise and take the repetitions more slowly to help you increase your strength. Keep your lower abdominals contracted throughout to focus the strengthening effect of the move and provide support for your lower back.

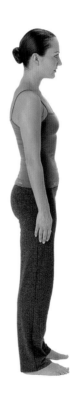

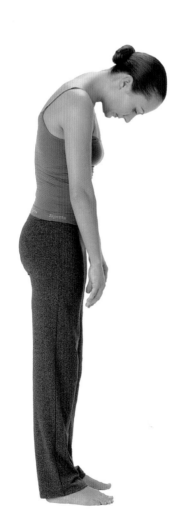

❶ Stand in neutral with your feet hip-width apart and your knees soft (slightly bent). Inhale and contract your lower abdominals; avoid hunching your shoulders or lifting your chest as you do this.

❸ Repeat Steps 1 and 2 of the previous version, this time keeping your legs straight, if possible, but without locking your knees, dropping your hands down to the floor.

❷ Exhale, drop your head forward, and start to roll down toward the floor using a slow, controlled movement.

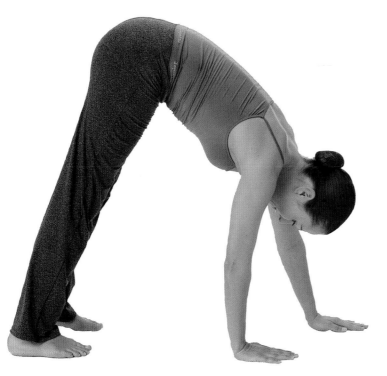

4 Still keeping your knees straight, as you exhale, walk your hands out away from your body until your body is parallel to the floor with your hands directly below your shoulders. Your toes should be tucked under, with your feet parallel. Focus on keeping your abdominals contracted; this will not only focus the strengthening effect of the exercise, but will also keep you from arching your back. Keep your eyes focused down toward the floor and keep continually lengthening along the back of your neck.

5 Inhale, then as you exhale, lower your upper body down until your nose almost touches the floor, keeping your elbows wide (pointing out slightly).

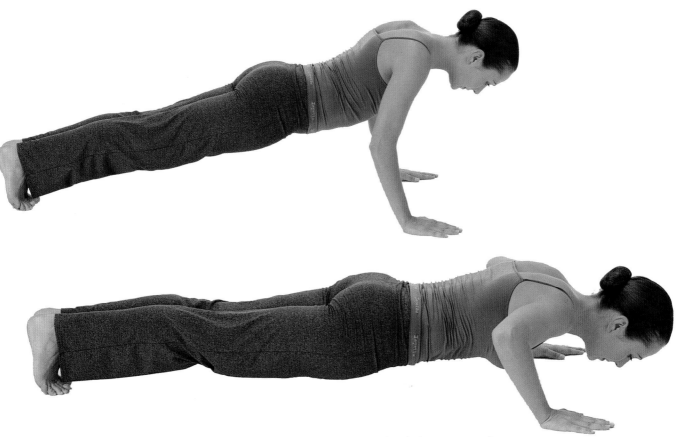

6 Repeat the Push-Up variation five to ten times. When you have finished, exhale as you walk your hands back, taking your weight back onto your feet and gently rolling back up through your spine to a standing position, bringing the head up last and lengthening out through the back of your neck and head toward the ceiling.

open leg rocker

intermediate

This exercise mobilizes your spine and builds strength in the abdominal area and your legs. If you find this exercise too difficult, try the Seal (pages 42–43) or Rolling Back (pages 38–39) moves instead. If your lower back is stiff, then keep working at the first level of this exercise until you have built up sufficient flexibility.

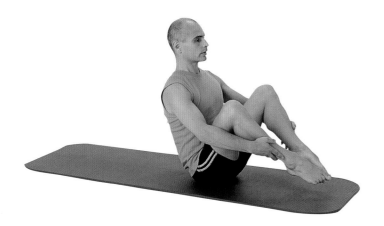

❶ Sit in an upright position with your legs in front of you, slightly apart, with knees bent and feet placed flat on the floor. Lengthen up through your spine and the back of your neck and draw the shoulder blades down and back. Place your hands on your ankles and lift your legs off the floor slightly, keeping your knees apart, but bringing your toes together. Find your point of balance, making sure you are keeping the length in your spine and neck. Focus your eyes directly in front of you and check that your weight is evenly spread across your buttocks—avoid leaning to one side.

❷ Inhale, and as you exhale, contract your abdominals, tilt your pelvis forward, and extend your left leg, keeping your knee soft and your toes gently pointed. The toes of the right foot stay in position, a few inches off the floor. You will need to concentrate on maintaining your balance as you extend your leg. When you first attempt this exercise, only extend your leg as far as you can without wobbling or losing your balance. At this stage, it is much more important for you to maintain the correct position than it is for you to fully straighten your leg. Once you have extended your leg as far as you can, inhale, exhale, contract your abdominals, tilt the pelvis, and bring your left leg back down to join your right leg.

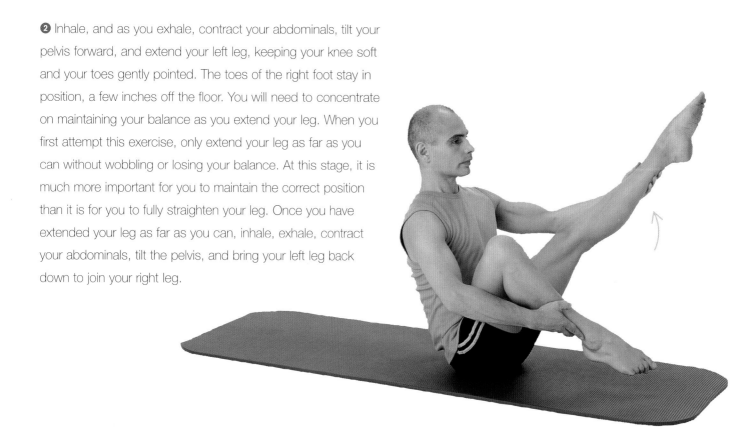

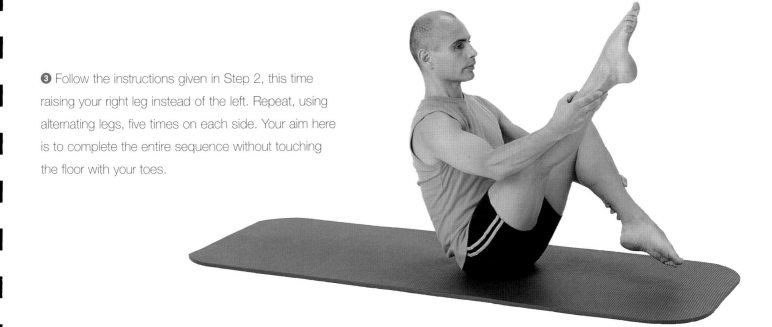

❸ Follow the instructions given in Step 2, this time raising your right leg instead of the left. Repeat, using alternating legs, five times on each side. Your aim here is to complete the entire sequence without touching the floor with your toes.

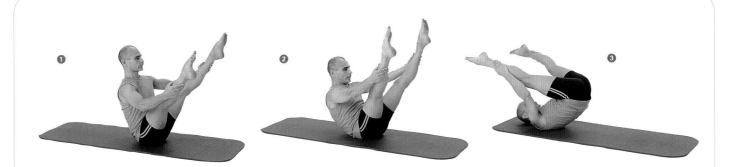

VARIATION: intermediate/advanced

❶ Follow the instructions given in Steps 1 and 2 above, this time extending first your left leg and then bringing the right up to join it, knees and feet apart, hands gently grasping the ankles. Inhale, then exhale, contract your abdominals, tilt the pelvis forward, and start to roll down onto the mat, vertebra by vertebra, in a smooth movement. Keep your legs straight, your spine lengthened, and your focus forward.

❷ Continue rolling back, bringing your legs over your head and keeping them at the same distance from your body throughout. If possible, your legs should be straight with your knees soft. If there is any tightness in your hamstrings, bend your legs a little. Avoid bringing your legs so far over your head that your feet touch the floor.

❸ Once you have reached your furthest point, inhale, contract your abdominals, and allow the momentum to help you rock back down through your spine, vertebra by vertebra, in a controlled, smooth movement. When you reach the starting position, inhale, exhale, contract your abdominals, tilt the pelvis forward, and continue with the rocking sequence. Repeat five to ten times. The whole exercise should be a controlled, continuous, flowing movement, using the momentum to help you. Avoid jerking your body as you bring your legs back over your head and roll down your spine to return to the starting position—use your abdominal muscles to control the move.

leg pull (supine)

advanced

The focus of this demanding exercise is to strengthen the abdominal core, your buttocks, your arms, and your shoulders. It also stretches the muscles of the chest and those of the upper legs. This move is contraindicated for anyone with wrist or shoulder problems.

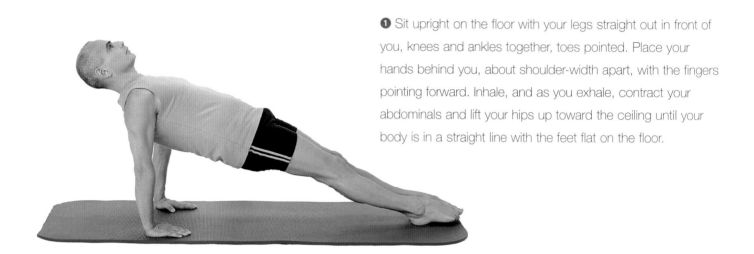

❶ Sit upright on the floor with your legs straight out in front of you, knees and ankles together, toes pointed. Place your hands behind you, about shoulder-width apart, with the fingers pointing forward. Inhale, and as you exhale, contract your abdominals and lift your hips up toward the ceiling until your body is in a straight line with the feet flat on the floor.

❷ Lengthen through your spine and drop the chin slightly toward the chest, keeping the back of your neck lengthened and making sure your shoulders are dropped down away from the ears. Focus your eyes forward.

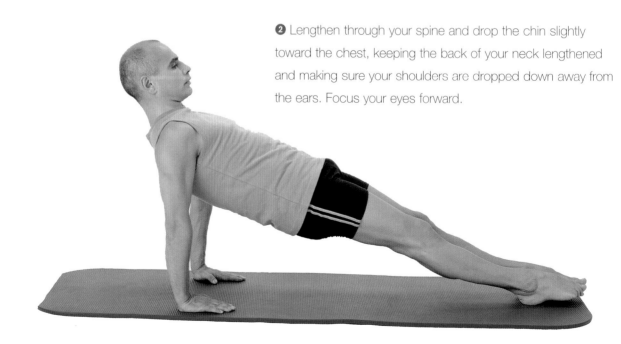

❸ Inhale, contract your abdominals, check that the back is in neutral, and raise your right leg toward the ceiling as you exhale. Keep the rest of your body in a line, avoiding dropping or lifting the hips as you raise your leg upward and continually lengthening your leg toward the ceiling. Push up from the heels of your hands to avoid sinking into the wrists or hunching your shoulders. Inhale, then exhale slowly and lower your right leg back down using a slow, controlled movement, placing the foot flat on the floor. Inhale and switch your weight onto this leg.

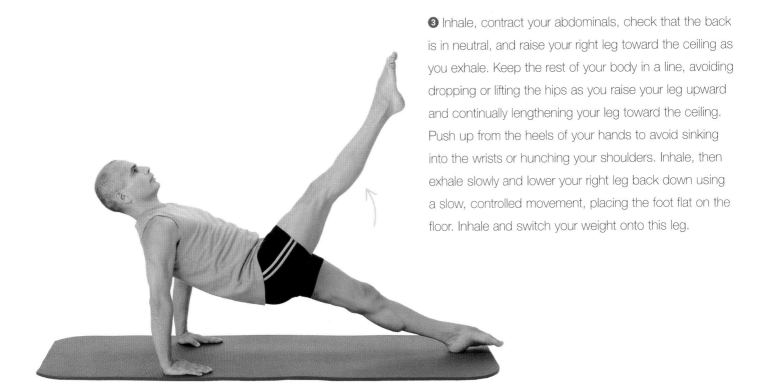

❹ Exhale and raise your left leg to the ceiling in the same way. Inhale with your leg extended to the ceiling and exhale as you lower your left leg back down to the floor. Repeat the sequence five to ten times on each side, alternating your legs each time.

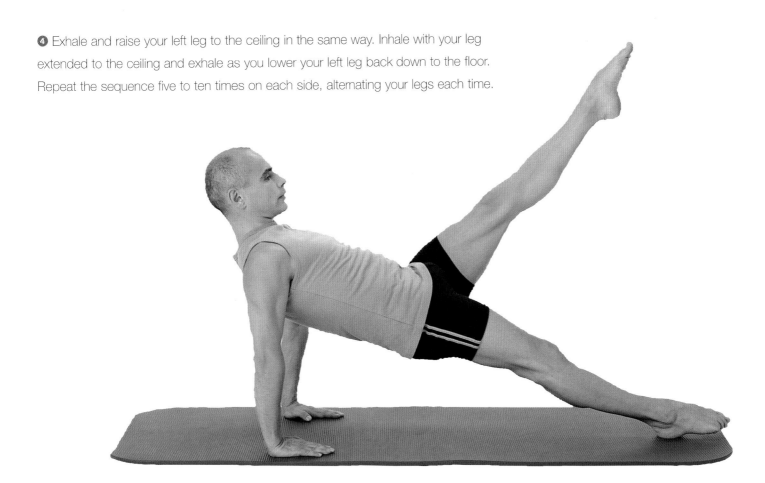

corkscrew

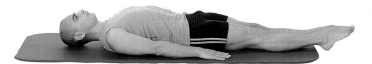
intermediate/advanced

This movement must only be attempted once you have built up enough strength in your abdominals and spine to maintain control even as you twist away from center with your legs and hips into an off-balance position.

1 Lie on your back with legs together and stretched straight out in front of you, toes pointing softly forward. Rest your arms by your sides, close to your body, palms facing downward.

2 Inhale, then exhale as you contract your abdominals and tilt your pelvis upward, raising your legs straight up away from the floor, keeping your spine in neutral.

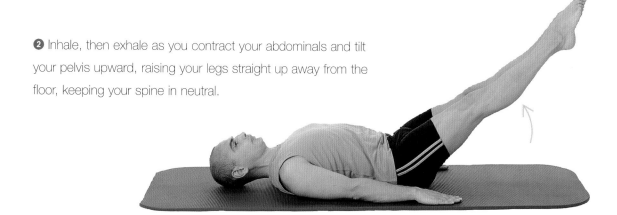

3 Continue to exhale as you bring your legs up and over your head, peeling your spine off the floor one vertebra at a time, gently squeezing the inner thighs together as you lift. The movement should be smooth and steady. Use your abdominal muscles to control the lift.

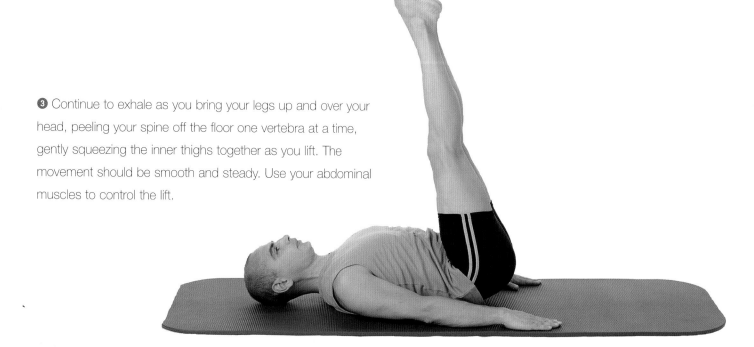

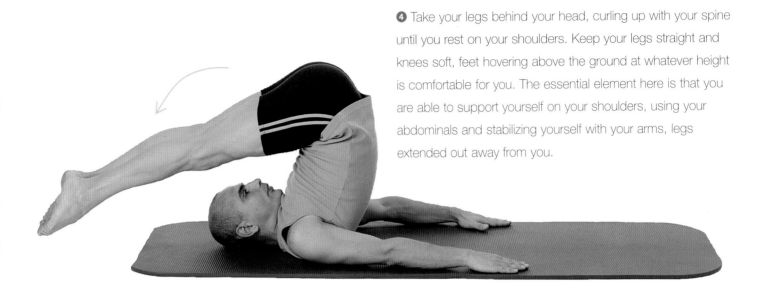

❹ Take your legs behind your head, curling up with your spine until you rest on your shoulders. Keep your legs straight and knees soft, feet hovering above the ground at whatever height is comfortable for you. The essential element here is that you are able to support yourself on your shoulders, using your abdominals and stabilizing yourself with your arms, legs extended out away from you.

❺ Inhale, then exhale, contract your abdominals, and as you continue to exhale, carry out the following movement. Keeping your legs and hips parallel, lower your body over to the right, using your arms to stabilize you. Slowly and evenly, draw a circle with the feet, moving them around to the right, then down, across, and upward to the left. Inhale, and as you exhale, reverse the movement, drawing the circle around to the left and down, across, and upward to the right, to complete the corkscrew motion. Repeat this motion a total of five to ten times. Inhale as you return to center and exhale as you roll your spine back down onto the floor and lower your legs to the starting position.

rolling into jackknife

intermediate/advanced

This move is a strength-building exercise that also works to open out your spine. It strengthens your abdominals and stretches the muscles of your back, shoulders, and neck. Make sure you keep your knees tucked in toward your chest as you roll backward onto the floor and use your abdominal muscles to bring you up into the jackknife position. This is an extremely challenging exercise; only attempt it once you have mastered the Rolling Back and Jackknife moves individually and are confident that your strength and muscle control are sufficiently developed.

❶ Sit upright on the floor with the heels raised, toes touching the ground, knees and ankles together, hands resting lightly on the outsides of the knees. Pull the shoulder blades down and back, and lengthen along the back of your neck. Inhale, contract your abdominals, and tilt the pelvis forward. Keep your eyes focused straight out in front of you.

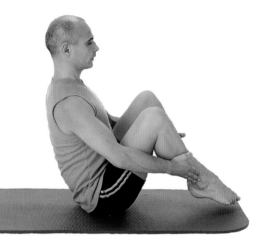

❷ Exhale, contract your abdominals, and roll back, bending your head slightly and tucking the chin in toward the chest, keeping the movement as slow and controlled as possible as you roll down vertebra by vertebra. Keep rolling back until your weight is balanced on the upper back and shoulder area.

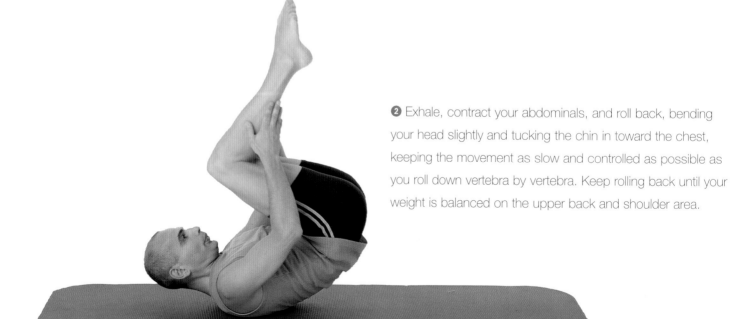

❸ Continue the movement, slowly extending your legs upward toward the ceiling to take you into the jackknife position. Squeeze the inner thighs together and squeeze your buttocks as you extend your legs. Keep your hands at the sides of your knees—your aim is to control the entire move with the abdominal core, without the aid of the hands and arm.

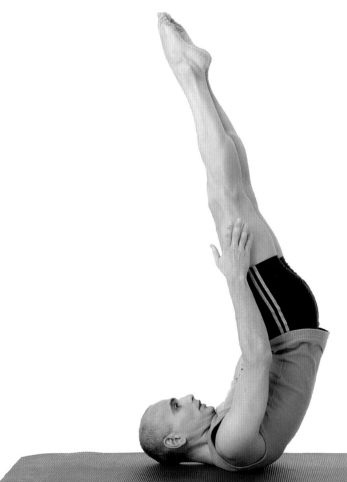

❹ Keep extending your legs until you are resting on your shoulders, neck, and arms with your body and legs in a straight line, pointing up toward the ceiling. Inhale, then exhale, contract your abdominals, and slowly roll back down through your spine, vertebra by vertebra, using a slow, even, controlled movement, keeping the feet positioned directly above your face for as long as possible. When you have rolled your spine back down to the floor as far as you can, keeping the feet in front of the face, lower your legs and bend your knees into your chest as you roll smoothly back to a balanced sitting position with your toes touching the floor once more. You will need to keep your abdominal muscles contracted and allow the momentum of the move to help bring you back to this position. Repeat five to ten times.

the roll over

intermediate/advanced

This movement improves the flexibility of your spine while strengthening your abdominals and improving muscle control. It also provides an intensive stretch to the hamstrings and stretches out the entire shoulder area. If you suffer from any neck or lower-back problems, avoid this exercise entirely.

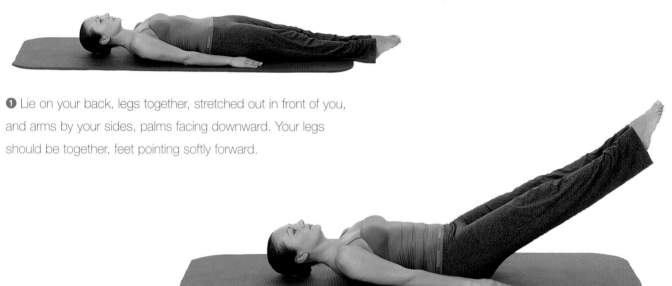

❶ Lie on your back, legs together, stretched out in front of you, and arms by your sides, palms facing downward. Your legs should be together, feet pointing softly forward.

❷ Inhale, then exhale and contract your abdominals as you start to raise your legs upward toward the ceiling, taking your legs apart slightly as you lift them and squeezing your buttocks. Press your hands into the floor, if necessary, to help you lift up and to give yourself stability.

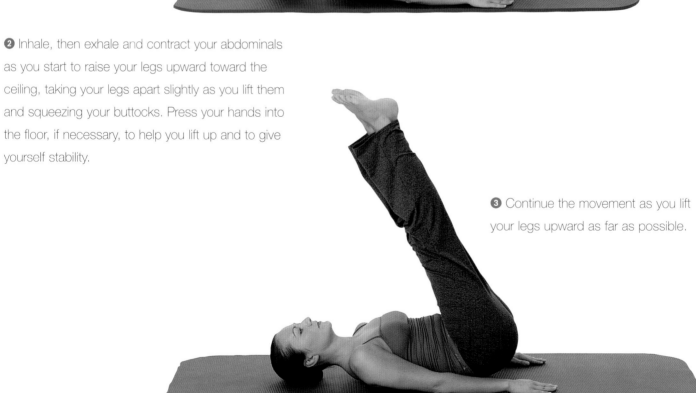

❸ Continue the movement as you lift your legs upward as far as possible.

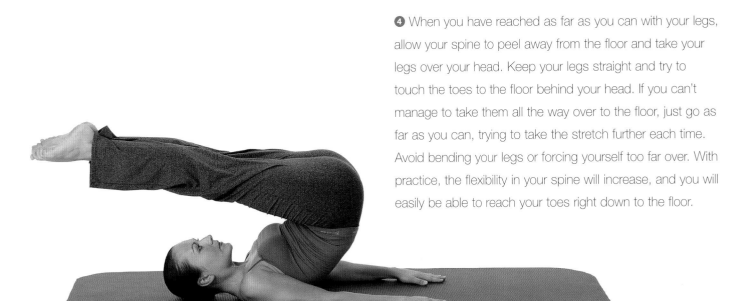

④ When you have reached as far as you can with your legs, allow your spine to peel away from the floor and take your legs over your head. Keep your legs straight and try to touch the toes to the floor behind your head. If you can't manage to take them all the way over to the floor, just go as far as you can, trying to take the stretch further each time. Avoid bending your legs or forcing yourself too far over. With practice, the flexibility in your spine will increase, and you will easily be able to reach your toes right down to the floor.

⑤ Inhale, then exhale, contract your abdominals once more, and start to roll back down, very slowly, vertebra by vertebra, using a controlled, even movement. Allow the abdominal muscles to bring you back down, all the while resisting the pull of gravity upon your body. Once your tailbone is in contact with the floor once more, bring your legs and feet together, keeping them a few inches above the ground, then inhale and repeat the sequence five to ten times in total.

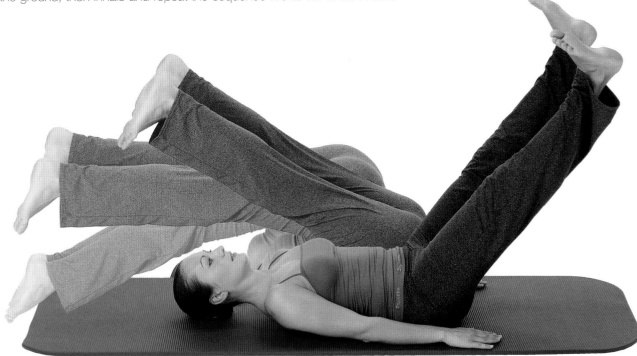

swan dive 1

beginner

This exercise works your abdominals, upper back, arms, and shoulders. It is essential that you keep lengthening through your spine and along the back of your neck throughout this exercise.

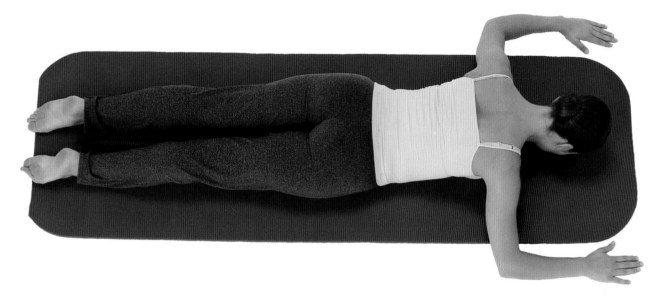

❶ Lie on your front, with your legs parallel, slightly apart, soles of the feet facing up to the ceiling. Your arms are positioned at shoulder height, elbows bent at a ninety-degree angle, with forearms in contact with the floor, palms down. Lengthen through the back of your neck, eyes looking straight down at the floor. Inhale, then as you exhale, contract your abdominals, and keeping the length in your spine and maintaining the lower back in neutral, lengthen up through the chest, allowing the upper body to lift off the ground very slightly. The forearms stay in contact with the floor throughout this movement. Inhale and lower your body back down. Repeat three to five times.

VARIATION 1

If you find it uncomfortable to keep your feet in the parallel position described above, try the movement positioning your legs so that the heels are dropped out to the sides with the big toes touching.

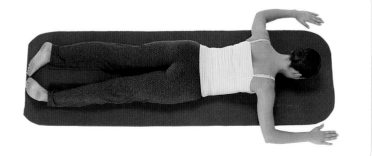

VARIATION 2: beginner/intermediate

This variation increases the stretch in the chest, arms, and upper back, and also engages the gluteals. Again, remember to keep lengthening through your spine and neck. The upper body is lifted and lengthened—avoid curving your body back as you lift, as this would cause pressure to the lower vertebrae. As for the initial level of this move, if your feet are uncomfortable in the parallel position, drop your heels out to the side, big toes touching.

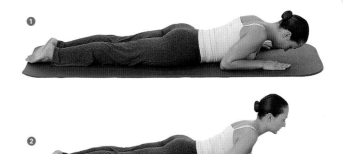

❶ Lie on your front with your legs parallel, slightly apart, soles of the feet facing upward. This time your arms are positioned close to your body, forearms in contact with the floor, palms placed on the floor on either side of your shoulders. Lengthen through your spine and the back of your neck, eyes looking down at the floor.

❷ Inhale, and as you exhale, contract your abdominals and lengthen up through the chest to lift the upper body off the ground, keeping the forearms in contact with the floor. While you do this, make sure you keep the length in your spine and maintain the lower back in neutral. When you have raised yourself as far as is comfortable, inhale and lower your body back down to the ground. Repeat five to ten times.

VARIATION 3: intermediate

This version of the Swan Dive is an extension of Variation 2. Here you allow your arms to extend, increasing the lift and stretch in the upper body, engaging the gluteals further and beginning to work the hamstrings. As in the other two variations, the heels may be dropped out to the side if the feet are not comfortable in the parallel position.

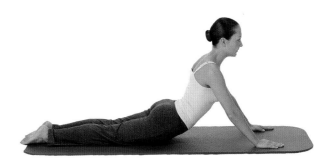

Follow the description for Variation 2, Step 1. Then inhale, and as you exhale, contract your abdominals and lengthen up through your chest and straighten your arms to lift the upper body off the floor. Keep your elbows soft and your arms bent very slightly. Focus on keeping the length through your spine as much as possible. your neck should be long and your eyes looking straight ahead. Make sure that your shoulders are dropped down and the shoulder blades pulled back and down. Inhale as you lower the upper body back down to the ground. Repeat five to ten times.

side bend **prone**

advanced

This exercise is a challenging development of the Side Bend Prep, strengthening the muscles and improving muscle control and general stability as you work to lift the weight of your body off the ground while maintaining your body alignment.

❶ Sit on your right side with your hips stacked one on top of the other. Extend your right leg, bend the left knee slightly, and cross the left foot over the right and place it flat down on the floor. Position your right hand on the floor directly beneath the right shoulder. Your arm should be straight, but avoid locking at the elbow. Let your left arm rest in front of your body, hand on the floor, palm upward. Eyes focus straight out throughout this sequence. Lengthen up through your spine and neck.

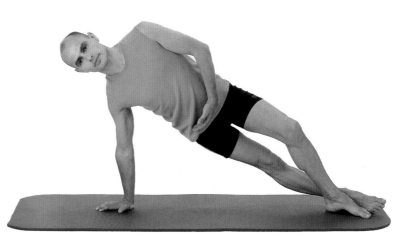

❷ Inhale, then exhale, contract your abdominals, and lift yourself up off the floor, pressing down with the left foot and the right hand. Keep your right arm straight, your left leg extended, and your spine and neck in a straight line. Your left arm should be curved, with the hand resting lightly just under the navel.

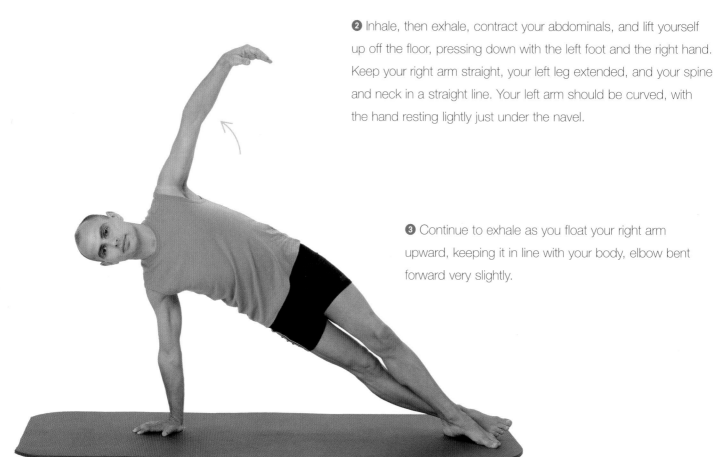

❸ Continue to exhale as you float your right arm upward, keeping it in line with your body, elbow bent forward very slightly.

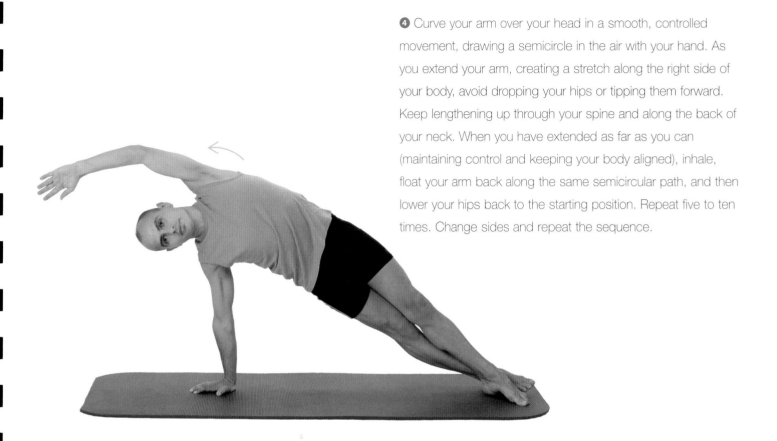

4 Curve your arm over your head in a smooth, controlled movement, drawing a semicircle in the air with your hand. As you extend your arm, creating a stretch along the right side of your body, avoid dropping your hips or tipping them forward. Keep lengthening up through your spine and along the back of your neck. When you have extended as far as you can (maintaining control and keeping your body aligned), inhale, float your arm back along the same semicircular path, and then lower your hips back to the starting position. Repeat five to ten times. Change sides and repeat the sequence.

VARIATION: advanced

This sequence is an addition to the above level, not a replacement for it. Once you have mastered the above technique and are confident in your ability to sustain a balanced position, keeping your body in alignment, continue with the following exercise.

1 Follow Steps 1 and 2, extending your arm so that your hand is pointing straight up to the ceiling, your eyes focused on your hand throughout the rest of the sequence. Keep the alignment of your body, and avoid tilting the uppermost hip backward. Inhale.

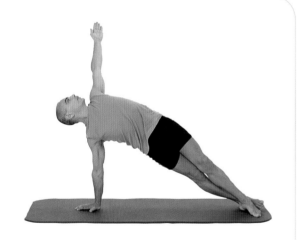

2 Contract your abdominals as you exhale and then start to curve your arm forward, keeping it at shoulder level and drawing a downward semicircle with your hand. Continue the movement using a slow, controlled motion, curving your hand down and through the gap beneath your right shoulder, creating a stretch across your shoulders and upper back. Take the movement as far as you can while maintaining the alignment of your body and maintaining your balance. Inhale as you draw your arm back along the same path, then inhale as you lower your body.

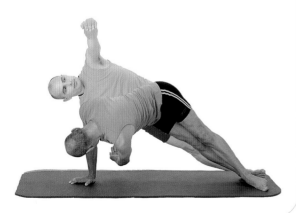

double leg kick

beginner/intermediate

This exercise works the back of your legs and your buttocks, while also providing a stretching to the front of your thighs. It also gives a gentle stretch to your upper back and shoulder area. If you suffer from any knee problems, substitute the kicking action with a slow stretching motion instead.

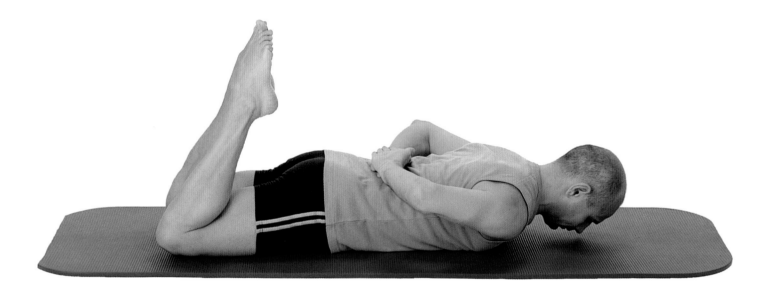

❶ Lie face down with your forehead touching the floor and your legs slightly apart. Place your hands behind your back, as far up toward your shoulder blades as you can without hunching your shoulders, palms positioned facing upward. Clasp the fingertips of the left hand with the right. Inhale slowly. Exhale, contract your abdominals, and extend your legs backward away from your body, pointing your toes and raising both legs approximately one inch away from the floor. Keeping your thighs in this raised position, press your hips into the floor, squeeze your inner thighs, and flick your heels toward your buttocks three times. Inhale and release your legs back down to the floor. Repeat the sequence ten times.

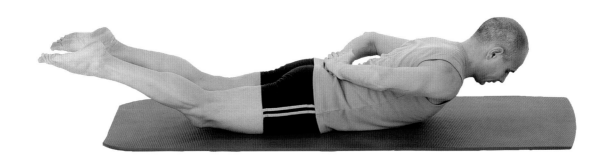

VARIATION 1: intermediate/advanced

This development involves raising your shoulders and extending your legs further. This increases the strengthening effect of the exercise on the upper back and also creates a stretch through the chest area. Keep your neck lengthened throughout the entire sequence.

Follow the instructions for Steps 1 and 2, stretching up through the chest to raise the upper body away from the floor as you extend your legs. Focus the eyes forward and down. As you extend your legs, lengthen them away from your body, allowing your thighs to lift away from the floor very slightly. Soften the knees so that the lower legs are raised a little higher than for the previous level. Keeping your thighs raised, press your hips into the floor, and flick your heels to your buttocks as for Step 2. Repeat the sequence ten times.

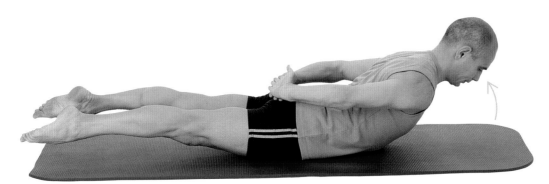

VARIATION 2: advanced

In this version, your legs are fully extended, creating a stretch through the hip joints and down through your legs and feet. Your shoulders are raised even higher to increase the strengthening effect on the upper body even further.

Follow the instructions for Steps 1 and 2, stretching up through the chest to raise the upper body away from the floor as far as you can. As you do this, allow your hands to slide down your back and come to rest on your tailbone. Your eyes should be focused forward and down. Keep lengthening along your spine and neck to avoid causing any pressure to the lower back. At the same time, fully extend your legs, lengthening them away from your body and allowing them to lift up toward the ceiling as high as possible while keeping the hips in contact with the floor. With your legs held in this position, with the hips pressed into the floor and the back arched slightly, flick the heels to your buttocks as for Step 2. Repeat the sequence ten times. Inhale as you release back down to the floor.

double leg stretch 2

intermediate/advanced

This exercise is a more advanced version of Double Leg Stretch 1 and requires a strong abdominal core. As you circle your arms, keep the contraction in your abdominals and the neutral position of the pelvis to help protect your lower back.

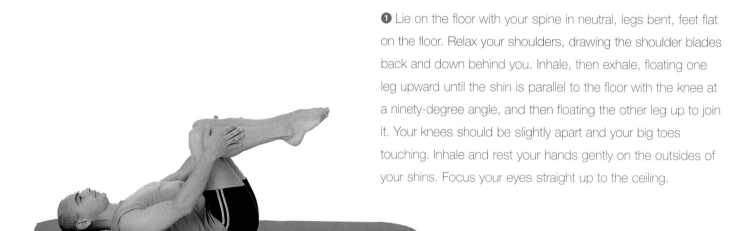

❶ Lie on the floor with your spine in neutral, legs bent, feet flat on the floor. Relax your shoulders, drawing the shoulder blades back and down behind you. Inhale, then exhale, floating one leg upward until the shin is parallel to the floor with the knee at a ninety-degree angle, and then floating the other leg up to join it. Your knees should be slightly apart and your big toes touching. Inhale and rest your hands gently on the outsides of your shins. Focus your eyes straight up to the ceiling.

❷ Keeping your spine in neutral and your hips level throughout the sequence, exhale, contract your abdominals, and bring your arms down toward the floor, then circle them out to the sides. At the same time, extend your legs slightly, keeping the knees bent and the toes softly pointed.

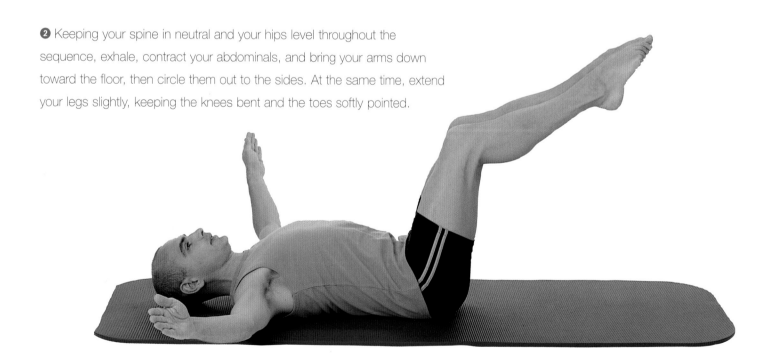

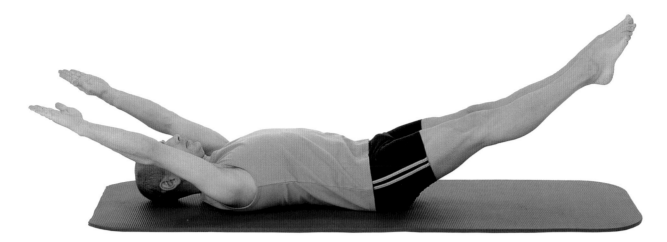

❸ Continue your arm movement, circling the lowered arms around until your hands are above your head, arms parallel, while extending your legs until they are straight. Avoid locking your knees. Keep your shoulders dropped and your shoulder blades drawn down and back. Inhale as you lift your arms up toward the ceiling and then bring them back down to shoulder level. At the same time, bring your legs back into your chest, knees apart, big toes together. Continue this sequence, circling your arms five to ten times. Change direction and circle your arms five to ten times in the other direction, exhaling as you take the parallel arms up and back (stretching away from your head) and extend your legs and inhaling as you circle your lowered arms out to the sides, down toward your body, and back up to the starting position, while at the same time bringing your legs in toward your chest.

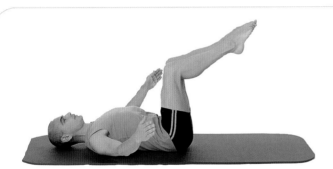

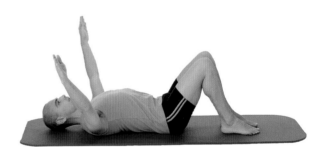

VARIATION: intermediate

If you experience any discomfort or tension in your lower back, adjust your leg position, raising your legs a little higher and drawing the knees in toward the chest. This will relieve any pressure in the lower back. If you are feeling any strain or soreness in your shoulders, decrease the size of your arm circles.

❶ Follow the instructions for Steps 1 and 2, but this time only extend your legs until they are at a right angle to your body, keeping your knees bent and your tailbone in

contact with the floor. Inhale and circle your arms up toward the ceiling, palms facing in, arms level with the shoulders.

❷ Exhale as you circle your arms out to the sides, taking them around and down to the sides. Keep circling as you inhale and raise them back up to shoulder level, lowering your legs to the floor. Repeat the sequence with your arms five to ten times. Keep your arms and shoulders relaxed, with the shoulder blades drawn down and back behind you.

swan dive 2

intermediate/advanced

This exercise strengthens and stretches your abdominals and upper body, and increases the strength in your arms. Keep lengthening through your spine and the back of your neck, and keep the contraction in your abdominals to prevent any pressure in your lower back.

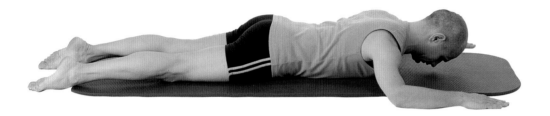

❶ Lie face down, with your legs parallel, slightly apart, soles of the feet upward. Your arms are positioned at shoulder height, elbows at a ninety-degree angle, forearms in contact with the floor, palms facing downward. Lengthen through the back of your neck, and keep looking straight down at the floor.

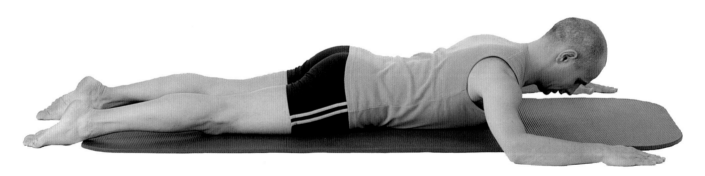

❷ Inhale, and as you exhale, contract your abdominals. Keeping the length in your spine and maintaining the lower back in neutral, lengthen up through the chest, allowing the upper body to lift off the ground, keeping the forearms in contact with the floor. Inhale and lower your body back down. Repeat three times, lifting the chest a little higher each time. Inhale, and as you exhale, lengthen up through your chest, lifting your upper body off the ground again, but this time also lifting your forearms and hands away from the ground very slightly so that they are no longer able to support you—now the work must all be done by your abdominals and chest muscles, intensifying the strengthening effect of this exercise. Inhale and lower your body and arms back down to the floor. Repeat five to ten times.

swan dive 3

advanced

This challenging version of the Swan Dive stretches and strengthens your abdominals, hip flexors, the front of your legs, your chest area, arms, spine, hamstrings, and gluteal muscles.

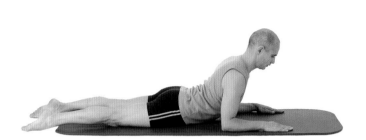

❶ Lie on your front, with your legs parallel, slightly apart, soles of the feet facing upward. This time your arms are positioned close to your body, forearms in contact with the floor, palms placed on the floor either side of your shoulders. Lengthen through your spine and along the back of your neck, eyes looking down and slightly forward. Inhale, then exhale, contracting the abdominal muscles, and lift up through your chest, keeping your forearms in contact with the floor.

❷ Continue the movement, straightening your arms and raising your upper body higher off the floor. Focus the eyes straight in front of you. Inhale and lower your upper body back down to the starting position.

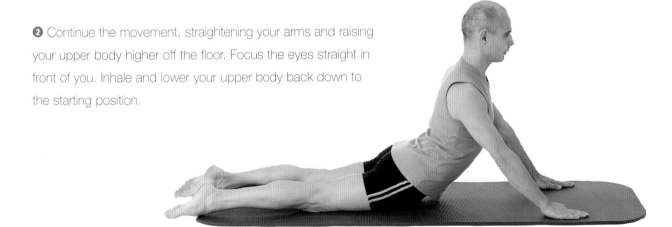

❸ Inhale, then exhale, contract your abdominals, tighten your buttocks a little, and raise your legs up off the ground, pressing your hips into the floor. Keep your eyes focused straight down, and concentrate on lengthening your spine and along the back of your neck. When you have lifted your legs as far as you are able, inhale and lower them back down to the floor. Repeat five to ten times.

side raises

The Side Raises work your abdominals, hips, buttocks, and leg muscles, strengthening your body and improving muscle control. Your back needs to be held in the neutral position with your spine lengthened and parallel to the floor throughout the whole exercise. Avoid tilting the uppermost hip and shoulder forward as your raise your legs.

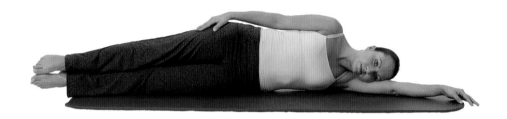

❶ Lie on your side with your body in a straight line, legs together. Your lower arm lies straight along the floor, supporting your head; the other arm rests along the side of your body in a relaxed position. Maintain neutral in this position, with your shoulders and hips in a line, and your back lengthened, lifting up at your waist to keep your spine parallel to the floor.

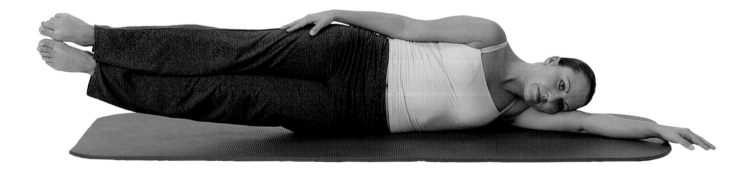

❷ Inhale, contract your abdominals, and holding your back in neutral, raise both legs up toward the ceiling as you exhale, keeping your legs in line with your body and squeezing your inner thighs together. The toes should be softly pointing down and away. Inhale and lower your legs back down, keeping your feet an inch or two above the floor. Repeat the lift five to ten times without touching the floor.

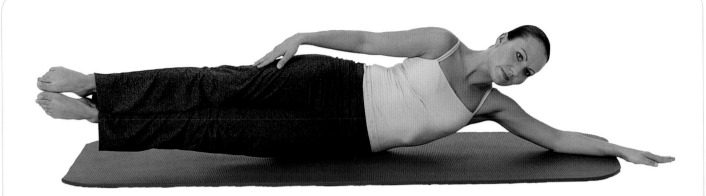

VARIATION: intermediate/advanced

This development increases the intensity of the move, stretching your waist and heightening the strengthening effect of the move by requiring your shoulders and hips to be raised simultaneously.

Repeat Step 1. Make sure that your back is maintained in the neutral position. Inhale, then exhale, contract your abdominals, and raise your shoulders up toward the ceiling at the same time as you lift your legs. Allow the uppermost hand to slide down the side of your body as you lift, keeping your shoulders down,

the shoulder blades pulled down and back, and your neck lengthened. Keep focusing your eyes straight in front of you. Inhale as you lower your shoulders and legs back down to the ground. Repeat the sequence five to ten times. If you experience any discomfort in the lower back or neck, then stop and return to the previous version. If you find that your muscles start to shake after a few lifts, decrease the number of repetitions—try to complete three repetitions to start with and then gradually build up to five and then ten.

hip flex

intermediate

This exercise provides an excellent stretch for the hip flexors, hamstrings, quadriceps, and gluteals, while also helping to improve your balance. Keep lengthening through your spine and the back of your neck as you work this sequence. Avoid twisting to one side or the other. Steps 2 to 5 are progressions of the basic Hip Flex move, each one at an increased level of difficulty, requiring improved muscle control and balance and slowly intensifying the stretch through the hip and thighs. Remember to use the exhalation each time to help you stretch. Hold each position for thirty to sixty seconds, allowing the stretch to gradually increase each time you exhale.

1 Position yourself with the feet together on the floor, knees bent and heels raised, hands placed either side of your feet, fingertips in contact with the floor.

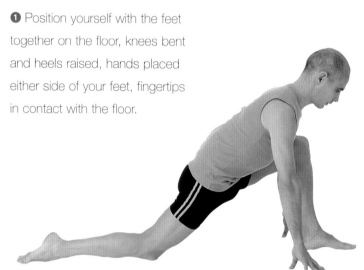

2 Inhale, contract your abdominals, and slide your right leg straight back behind you as you exhale, making sure that it stays in line with your hip. Place your right knee on the floor and lengthen your body forward over your left leg, bringing the left knee over your left ankle, to create a stretch through the front of the right thigh, the hips, and the left thigh. Keep the eyes focused forward and down, and continually lengthen along the back and your neck.

TIP

With this move, you can choose how far to take this sequence. By all means, complete the whole sequence, if you are able, but if you prefer, then just take the exercise as far as you can. However, you must always start with Step 1 and work through the steps in the order they are given here.

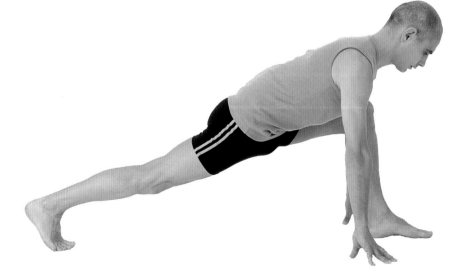

3 Inhale, tuck the toes of the right foot under, and raise your right knee off the floor to create a stretch through the hamstring at the back of your right leg and increase the stretch through the front of the thigh. Exhale and increase this stretch slightly, pressing down toward the floor with the right heel.

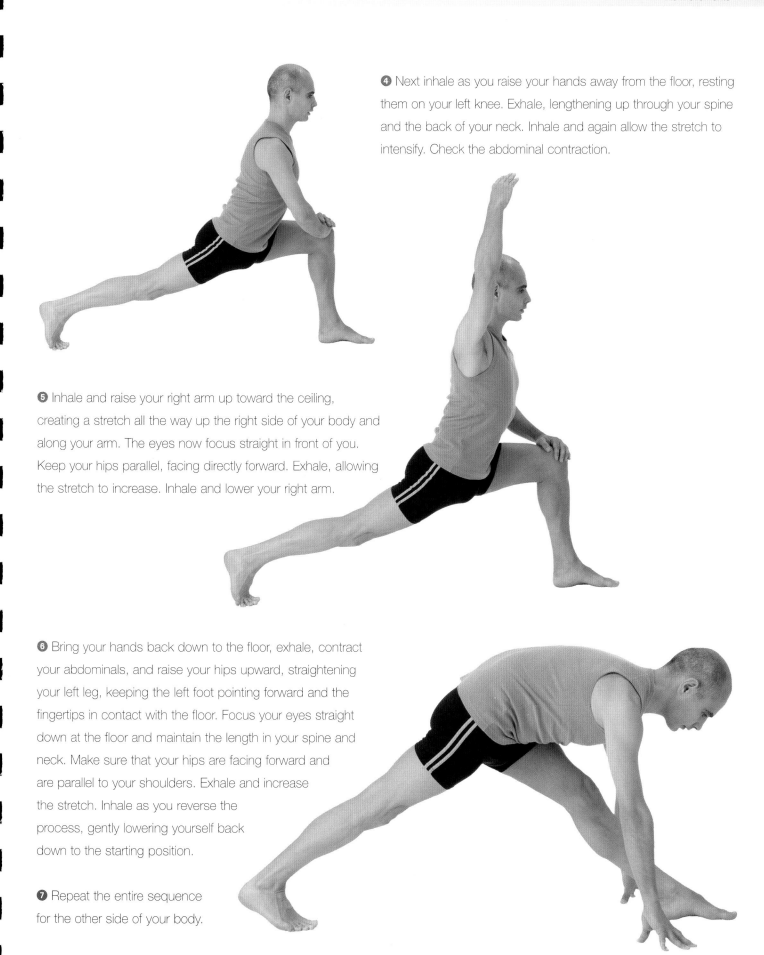

❹ Next inhale as you raise your hands away from the floor, resting them on your left knee. Exhale, lengthening up through your spine and the back of your neck. Inhale and again allow the stretch to intensify. Check the abdominal contraction.

❺ Inhale and raise your right arm up toward the ceiling, creating a stretch all the way up the right side of your body and along your arm. The eyes now focus straight in front of you. Keep your hips parallel, facing directly forward. Exhale, allowing the stretch to increase. Inhale and lower your right arm.

❻ Bring your hands back down to the floor, exhale, contract your abdominals, and raise your hips upward, straightening your left leg, keeping the left foot pointing forward and the fingertips in contact with the floor. Focus your eyes straight down at the floor and maintain the length in your spine and neck. Make sure that your hips are facing forward and are parallel to your shoulders. Exhale and increase the stretch. Inhale as you reverse the process, gently lowering yourself back down to the starting position.

❼ Repeat the entire sequence for the other side of your body.

cancan

intermediate/advanced

The Cancan focuses on strengthening the abdominal muscles and the back, and stretching and strengthening your legs and hip joints. Concentrate on making the movement as flowing as possible, keeping it slow and controlled throughout. Press down with the heels of the hands to avoid collapsing at the wrists.

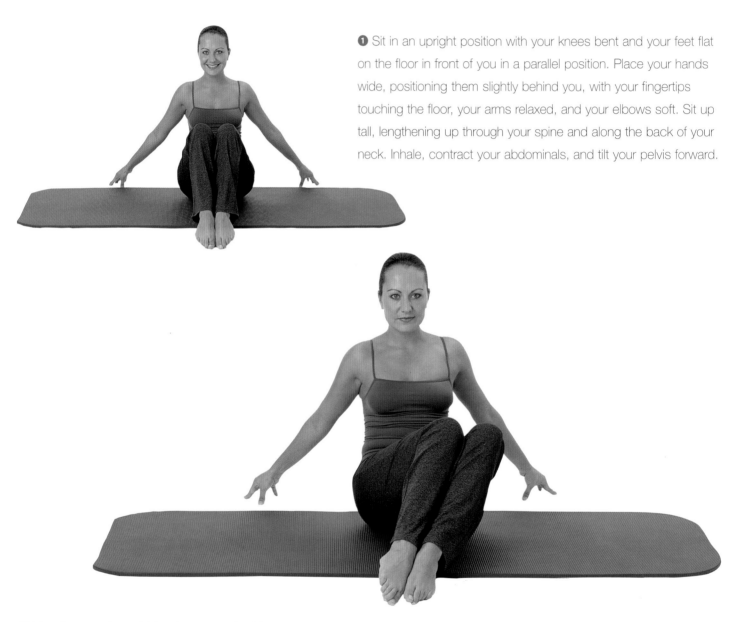

❶ Sit in an upright position with your knees bent and your feet flat on the floor in front of you in a parallel position. Place your hands wide, positioning them slightly behind you, with your fingertips touching the floor, your arms relaxed, and your elbows soft. Sit up tall, lengthening up through your spine and along the back of your neck. Inhale, contract your abdominals, and tilt your pelvis forward.

❷ Keeping your inner thighs, knees, and ankles pressed together, raise your heels up off the ground so that only your toes are touching the ground. Exhale as you contract your abdominals and lower your knees over to the left, keeping the hips level and both buttocks in contact with the floor. Take the knees as far over as you can while maintaining your body position. Inhale as you bring your legs back up to center and exhale as you take them over to the right. Repeat five to ten times.

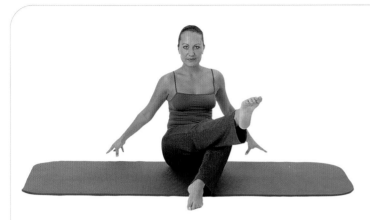

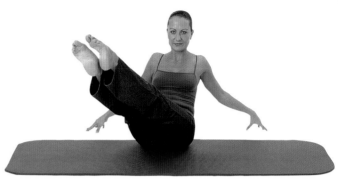

VARIATION 1: intermediate/advanced

This development further stretches your leg as you extend it out away from your body and also works to improve balance and coordination.

Follow the instructions for Step 1. Raise your heels off the ground so that only your toes are touching the ground. Exhale, contract your abdominals, and extend your left leg out away from your body as you drop your knees to the right, squeezing your thighs together. Keep your hips level and both buttocks in contact with the floor. Inhale as you bring your legs back to center, lowering the left foot back down to the floor. Repeat, this time extending your right leg and lowering over to the left. Repeat the sequence five to twenty times, keeping the movement as flowing and controlled as possible.

VARIATION 2: advanced

This variation is similar to the previous level, but extending both legs out. It requires a great deal of strength and muscle control in your abdominals. Make sure that you are fully confident with the first variation before you attempt this challenging move. If you feel any discomfort in your lower back or find you are unable to hold the position, then you need to return to the previous levels until you have built up more strength and control.

Follow the instructions for Variation 1, this time extending both legs out away from your body and over to the left in one smooth movement as you exhale. Curl back a little as you raise your legs up off the ground to find your position of balance, and use your fingertips to stabilize you, keeping your elbows soft. Inhale as you bend your knees and lower your legs back to center, touching the floor briefly with the toes, then exhale as you extend your legs out and over to the right, inhaling as you bring them back to center once more. Repeat five to ten times.

glute stretch

intermediate/advanced

You should follow any sequence of strengthening exercises by stretching the muscles you have been working. The Glute Stretch is an excellent move to include after doing any leg lifts. It stretches out the gluteal muscles and the lower back and helps to open up the hip area. This exercise can be particularly helpful to anyone suffering from any tightness in the lower back.

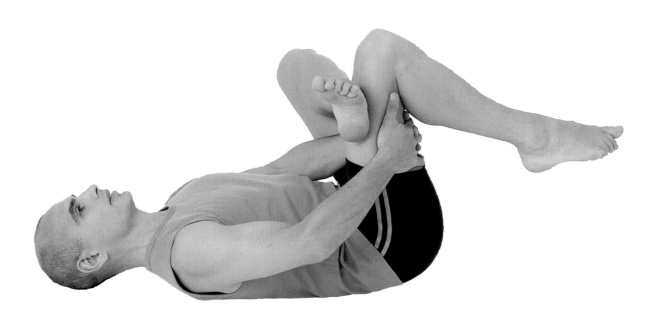

❶ Lie on your back in the neutral position, with your legs bent and your arms by your sides. Inhale and float your legs up toward your chest, one at a time, knees bent, and then cross your left ankle over your right knee. Clasp your hands around your right knee. Focus your eyes straight up to the ceiling.

❷ Exhale, lengthen your spine and neck, contract your abdominals, and ease your right thigh in toward your chest with your hands to create a stretch in your left leg. Inhale and exhale three to five times, trying to draw your leg in closer to the chest each time to increase the stretch. Inhale and release your legs back to the starting position.

❸ Repeat on the other side. If you feel any pain or discomfort in your lower back, release your right leg a little—you may be working your legs too hard. If the discomfort continues, stop.

VARIATION: intermediate
If you are finding it too difficult to keep your ankle in position across the opposite knee, try moving the ankle further up the opposite thigh, closer to your torso.

inner thigh stretch

intermediate/advanced

This gentle stretch relieves tightness and releases tension in the muscles of the inner thigh. It also helps to rebalance the pelvis as it works to stretch both sides of your body equally. This is essentially a passive exercise that uses gravity to create the stretch. Pressing down on the inner thighs intensifies this stretch, but avoid pressing too hard and risking overstretching your muscles. Remember to work in time with the breath as you slowly press down on the knees.

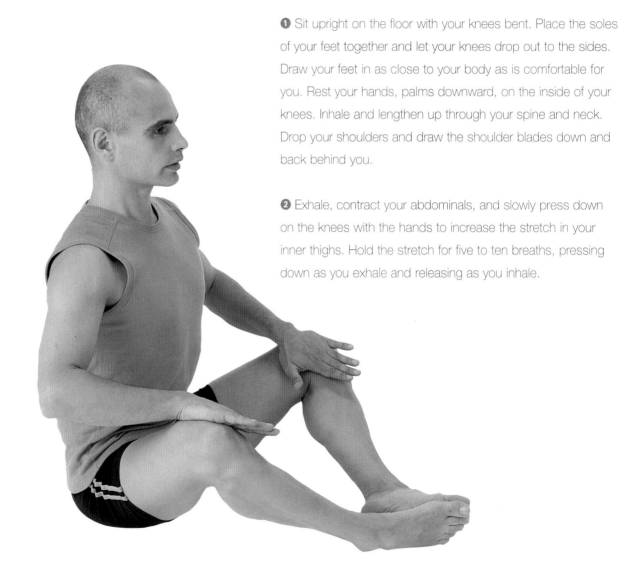

❶ Sit upright on the floor with your knees bent. Place the soles of your feet together and let your knees drop out to the sides. Draw your feet in as close to your body as is comfortable for you. Rest your hands, palms downward, on the inside of your knees. Inhale and lengthen up through your spine and neck. Drop your shoulders and draw the shoulder blades down and back behind you.

❷ Exhale, contract your abdominals, and slowly press down on the knees with the hands to increase the stretch in your inner thighs. Hold the stretch for five to ten breaths, pressing down as you exhale and releasing as you inhale.

VARIATION: intermediate

If you are uncomfortable sitting in this position, sit on the edge of a cushion or a folded towel to raise yourself up off the floor a little.

standing pecs stretch

intermediate

This exercise appears to be very simple but actually provides an intensive stretch to the pectoral muscles and your shoulders, while also opening out the chest and creating a stretch across the back of your neck. Make sure your weight is evenly distributed over both feet and avoid swaying or leaning forward or back as you stretch your arms. This is an excellent stretch for anyone who spends a great deal of time sitting at a computer or behind the wheel of a vehicle.

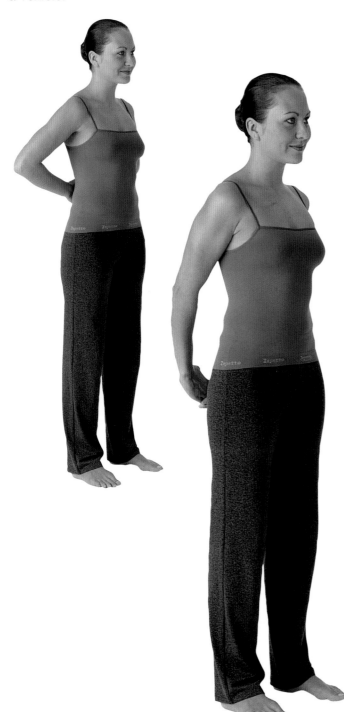

❶ Stand with your feet parallel, hip-width apart, knees soft, and arms by your sides. Lengthen up through your spine and neck, and focus the eyes forward, directly in front of you. Drop your shoulders and draw the shoulder blades down and back. Inhale and contract your abdominals as you take your arms behind you, grasping the fingers of one hand with the other. Exhale and take the hands up your spine as far as you can, keeping them close in to your body. Avoid hunching your shoulders or rounding them forward as you raise the hands. Hold for three to five breaths, increasing the stretch a little further on each breath out. Inhale and release your arms back down.

❷ Exhale as you bring the hands down behind you as far as possible, dropping your shoulders down, but keeping your body alignment and avoiding leaning back. Hold for three to five breaths, again trying to increase the stretch a little each time you exhale. Inhale and release your arms back down. Repeat the sequence five to ten times.

chair pecs stretch

intermediate/advanced

These two moves stretch out the shoulder muscles and open out the chest, helping to relieve any tension in the upper body. Keep the hips level throughout and your spine in neutral—avoid dropping at your waist as you stretch your shoulders downward.

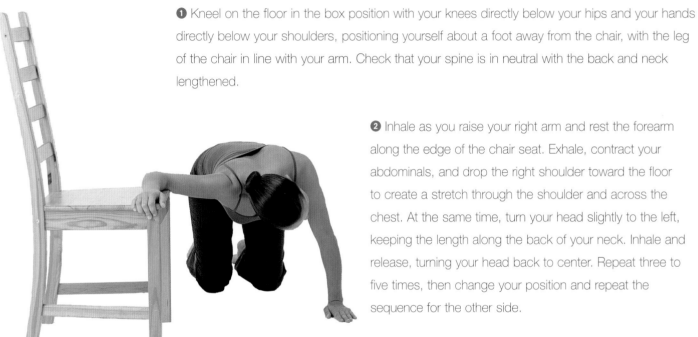

❶ Kneel on the floor in the box position with your knees directly below your hips and your hands directly below your shoulders, positioning yourself about a foot away from the chair, with the leg of the chair in line with your arm. Check that your spine is in neutral with the back and neck lengthened.

❷ Inhale as you raise your right arm and rest the forearm along the edge of the chair seat. Exhale, contract your abdominals, and drop the right shoulder toward the floor to create a stretch through the shoulder and across the chest. At the same time, turn your head slightly to the left, keeping the length along the back of your neck. Inhale and release, turning your head back to center. Repeat three to five times, then change your position and repeat the sequence for the other side.

VARIATION: advanced

This version gives a more intensive stretch to the pectoral muscles. Do not attempt it if you suffer from any knee problems.

Kneel in front of the chair in the box position. Again, your knees should be hip-width apart, with your feet parallel. Check that your spine is in neutral, then inhale as you lift one hand at a time and rest it on the seat of the chair. Focus your eyes straight down at the floor. Exhale and lower your shoulders toward the floor, keeping the back in neutral with the hips level.

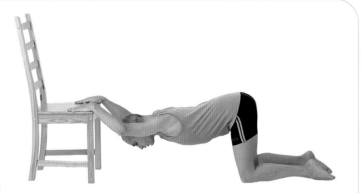

Hold for three to five breaths, trying to increase the stretch with each breath out. Inhale and release your shoulders back up. Repeat the sequence a total of five to ten times.

foam roller

intermediate/advanced

This exercise is carried out using a special type of foam roller. The roller needs to be firm enough to support your spine and allow you to balance. This move increases your balance, core strength, stability, and muscle control. Build up this sequence step-by-step, according to your muscle control and balance.

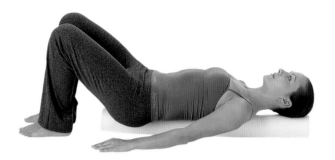

❶ Lie on the floor with the foam roller supporting your spine and head. Place your knees and feet on the floor, hip-width apart, and relax your arms down by your sides. Focus your eyes straight up at the ceiling.

❷ Inhale and float your arms up away from the floor an inch or two. Exhale, contract your abdominals, and lengthen your arms away from you, stretching down through your shoulders and drawing the shoulder blades back behind you. Use the abdominal contraction to keep your body stable and avoid rolling to one side or the other. Hold this position for three to five breaths, increasing the stretch each time you exhale. Inhale and lower your arms back down to the floor.

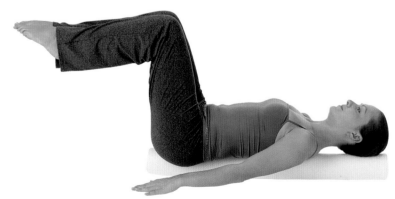

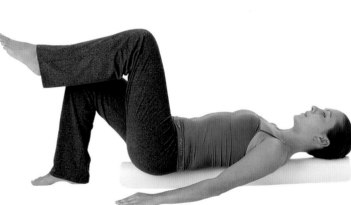

❸ Exhale and float your left leg up until the shin is parallel with the floor. Inhale and lower your leg back to the floor. Keep the hips level and your right leg stable, avoiding rolling to the side as you lift the other leg. Do the same for your right leg. Repeat the sequence slowly five to ten times, alternating your legs each time.

❹ Follow the instructions for Step 3, this time floating both legs up, one at a time, and lengthening your arms away from the floor as you find your point of balance.

climb tree

advanced

This advanced exercise requires a great deal of core strength and muscle control. Use your abdominals to allow you to roll up off the ground and make sure you maintain the alignment of your body as you stretch. It is much more important for you to work slowly, keeping control and stability, rather than pushing yourself to take the stretch further than you are able and struggling with the exercise.

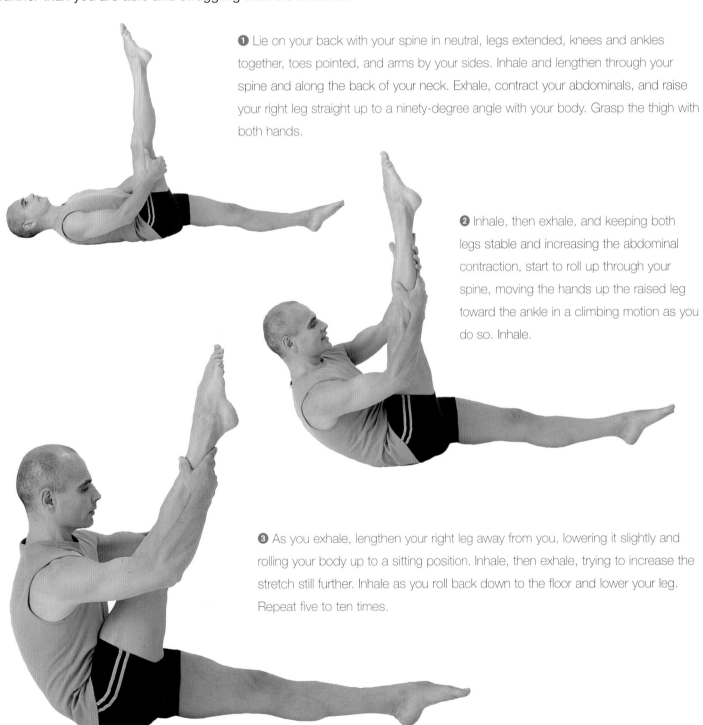

❶ Lie on your back with your spine in neutral, legs extended, knees and ankles together, toes pointed, and arms by your sides. Inhale and lengthen through your spine and along the back of your neck. Exhale, contract your abdominals, and raise your right leg straight up to a ninety-degree angle with your body. Grasp the thigh with both hands.

❷ Inhale, then exhale, and keeping both legs stable and increasing the abdominal contraction, start to roll up through your spine, moving the hands up the raised leg toward the ankle in a climbing motion as you do so. Inhale.

❸ As you exhale, lengthen your right leg away from you, lowering it slightly and rolling your body up to a sitting position. Inhale, then exhale, trying to increase the stretch still further. Inhale as you roll back down to the floor and lower your leg. Repeat five to ten times.

chest stretch

Rubber exercise bands are a useful addition to certain Pilates exercises and are available from specialty suppliers. If you do not have a band, use a rolled-up towel or scarf, although they do not work as well, as they do not have the same elasticity. Keep your spine in neutral and your shoulders dropped throughout these movements.

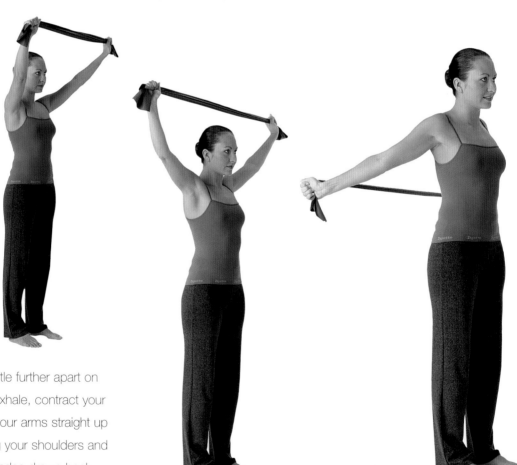

❶ Stand with your feet parallel, hip-width apart. Lengthen along your spine and neck and draw the shoulder blades back down behind you. Grasp the band with both hands, approximately eighteen inches apart, holding it out in front of you. Inhale, then as you exhale, contract your abdominals and move the hands apart and back together, stretching and releasing the band in a fairly rapid motion. This works your arms and stretches the chest. Stretch and release three times as you exhale, three times as you inhale. Repeat the sequence five to ten times.

❷ Move the hands a little further apart on the band. Inhale, then exhale, contract your abdominals, and raise your arms straight up in front of you, dropping your shoulders and keeping the shoulder blades drawn back and down.

❸ Continue the movement, taking your arms over your head, arms straight, elbows soft. As you start to take your arms over behind your head, allow the hands to move further apart, creating tension in the band.

❹ Take your arms all the way over as far as you can, then inhale and slowly bring your arms back, using a smooth, controlled motion. Repeat ten times, exhaling as you circle your arms back and inhaling as you bring them forward.

hamstring stretch

intermediate

The aim of this exercise is to stretch the hamstrings while keeping the correct alignment and avoiding creating tension in any other part of your body. Stretching your hamstrings and releasing any tightness can greatly improve the posture and your body's overall flexibility.

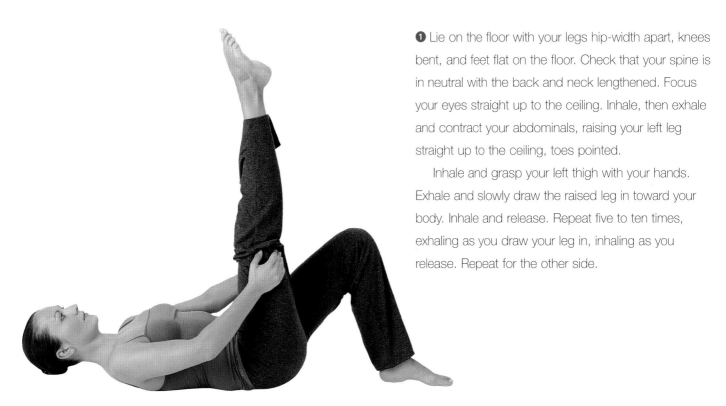

❶ Lie on the floor with your legs hip-width apart, knees bent, and feet flat on the floor. Check that your spine is in neutral with the back and neck lengthened. Focus your eyes straight up to the ceiling. Inhale, then exhale and contract your abdominals, raising your left leg straight up to the ceiling, toes pointed.

Inhale and grasp your left thigh with your hands. Exhale and slowly draw the raised leg in toward your body. Inhale and release. Repeat five to ten times, exhaling as you draw your leg in, inhaling as you release. Repeat for the other side.

VARIATION: intermediate/advanced

For these two variations, you need to use an exercise band (or a small towel) to intensify the stretch to the back of your leg. Keep both hips in contact with the floor as you stretch.

Follow Step 1 above, bringing the knee into the chest to place the band around the foot and then extending your leg up to the ceiling, keeping the foot flexed. Exhale, contract your abdominals, and pull the band in toward you to increase the flex in the foot and give a stronger stretch to the hamstrings. Keep your shoulders dropped and your elbows in contact with the floor. Inhale and release. Repeat five to ten times, exhaling as you draw your leg in, inhaling as you release. Repeat for the other side.

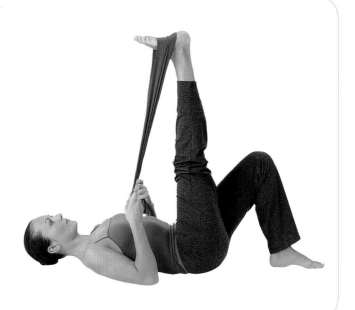

chest stretch

intermediate/advanced

The ring is another practical piece of equipment that enhances the effect of certain Pilates moves. As you exercise, it provides extra resistance for you to work against, increasing the strengthening effect of the movements.

❶ Sit cross-legged on the floor and lengthen up through your spine and neck. Keep your shoulders dropped and your elbows fairly close to your body as you hold the ring in front of you, between the palms of your hands. Inhale, then exhale, contract your abdominals, and squeeze the palms together. Inhale and release. Repeat ten times using a slow, even motion in time with your breath.

❷ Lift the ring above your head and repeat the squeezing movement described in Step 1. Keep your shoulders down and the shoulder blades pulled back and down behind you.

❸ Holding the ring in front of you again, repeat the sequence once more, this time twisting at your waist to take the ring to the side. Do ten squeezes on one side, then inhale and bring your body back to center. Twist around to the other side for another ten squeezes. Inhale and release back to center.

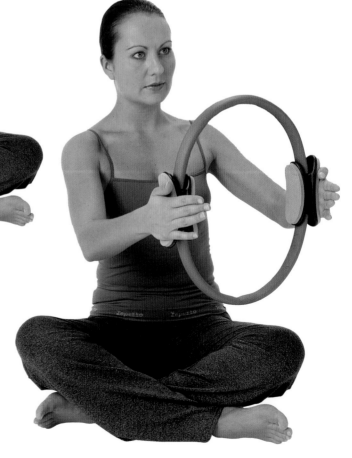

triceps stretch **(with ring)**

advanced

The aim of this exercise is to push down with the hands as far as possible, to stretch your triceps while maintaining your body in the neutral position. If you start to feel any strain in the chest or neck or cannot maintain the position, then you are working too hard—only push as far as you can with ease.

❶ Lie on the floor with your spine in neutral, your back and neck lengthened, knees bent and feet hip-width apart. Inhale and place the ring on the floor above your head and hold it in position with the palms of your hands.

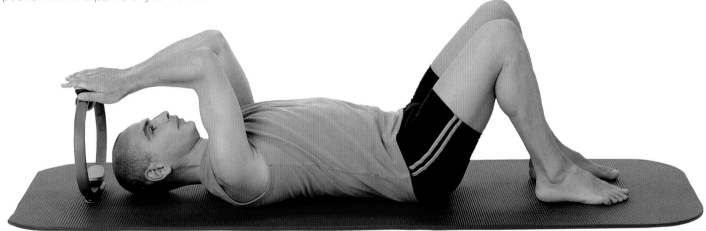

❷ Exhale, contract your abdominals, and press the ring into the floor as much as you can while holding your body in alignment. The forearms should be parallel, with your elbows pointing up to the ceiling. Make sure your shoulders are dropped away from the ears, and keep the knees stable—don't let them lean to one side. Check that the hips are level and your abdominals are contracted. Inhale as you release the pressure on the hands. Repeat ten times, exhaling as you press down on the ring and inhaling as you release.

the hundred (with ring)

intermediate/advanced

This is a variation on the Hundred described on pages 40–41. Using the ring to do this move stabilizes your legs in position and also increases the work in your legs as they squeeze inward against the ring.

❶ Place the ring between your ankles and then position yourself on the floor with your legs extended. Rest your arms by your sides with palms facing downward. Your spine should be in neutral. Inhale, contract your lower abdominals, and exhale, lifting the extended legs up to an angle of forty-five degrees. Holding your legs in this position, drop your shoulders and lengthen your arms, lifting and lowering using a pulsing action—five times as you inhale and five times as you exhale—until you reach one hundred. Squeeze your ankles together as you pulse your arms. Keep your eyes focused on the ceiling.

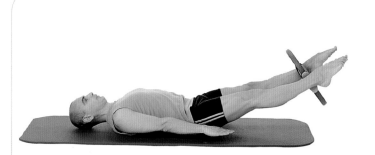

VARIATION 1: advanced

To give yourself a greater challenge and increase the intensity of the exercise in the abdominal area, follow the sequence described above, but with your legs lowered down toward the floor. If you find you cannot hold the alignment or your muscles start to tire, raise your legs again as you continue to pulse your arms.

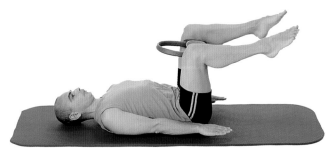

VARIATION 2: beginner/intermediate

In this version, the squeeze occurs with the inner thighs rather than with your ankles. Start with the knees bent, feet flat on the floor. Raise both legs, one at a time, and place the ring between your knees. Keep your legs at right angles to your body and make sure both hips stay in contact with the floor. Relax and lengthen your neck as you pulse.

single leg press **(with ring)**

intermediate/advanced

This movement is excellent for strengthening your leg muscles and improving stamina. Lengthen up through your spine and neck as you exercise, keeping your torso upright and the shoulder blades pulled back and down. Extend the lowered leg as much as you can as you press with the other leg.

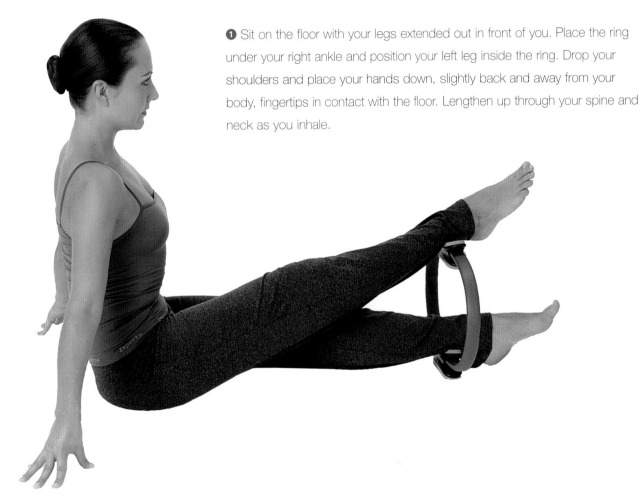

❶ Sit on the floor with your legs extended out in front of you. Place the ring under your right ankle and position your left leg inside the ring. Drop your shoulders and place your hands down, slightly back and away from your body, fingertips in contact with the floor. Lengthen up through your spine and neck as you inhale.

❷ Exhale and contract your abdominals. As you continue to exhale, press down on the ring with your right leg while at the same time lengthening your left leg away from you. Keep the hips stable and in contact with the floor at all times. Repeat the press ten to twenty times, exhaling as you press down and inhaling as you release. Try to increase the pressure on the ring with your right ankle with each exhalation. The eyes should be focused directly in front of you for the entire sequence; this will help you to maintain your posture and keep you from losing your balance.

❸ Change position and repeat for the other side. If you find that your leg muscles begin to shake or you can no longer maintain the position, then reduce the number of repetitions for the time being, until your strength and stamina increases.

swan dive **with ball**

intermediate/advanced

Exercise balls vary in size and you need to choose the one that is appropriate for your build. For this particular exercise you need to be able to position yourself comfortably over the ball while kneeling on the floor. The advantage of using the ball for this move is to increase the stretch through your back as you curve forward.

❶ Kneel on the floor with your knees and ankles together. Curve your body over the exercise ball and place your hands just behind your ears, elbows pointing outward. Inhale in this position, with the head dropped very slightly toward the floor.

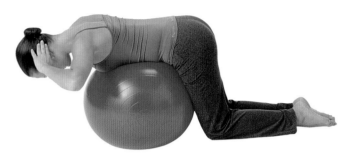

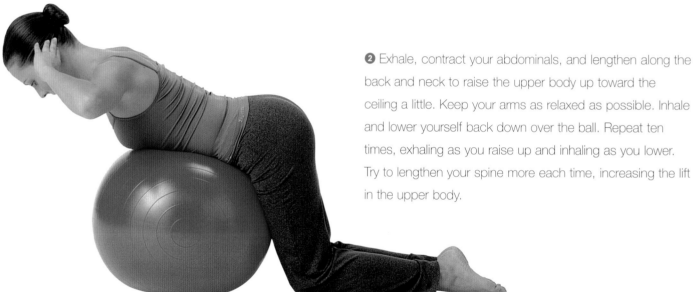

❷ Exhale, contract your abdominals, and lengthen along the back and neck to raise the upper body up toward the ceiling a little. Keep your arms as relaxed as possible. Inhale and lower yourself back down over the ball. Repeat ten times, exhaling as you raise up and inhaling as you lower. Try to lengthen your spine more each time, increasing the lift in the upper body.

VARIATION: advanced

Keeping your arms down by your sides increases the lengthening effect of your spine, intensifying the strengthening effect of this exercise upon your back and shoulder muscles.

Follow the instructions given in Steps 1 and 2 above, but this time place your arms down by your sides and keep lengthening them away, stretching down through your shoulders as you lift and lower the upper body. Repeat the sequence ten times, as above.

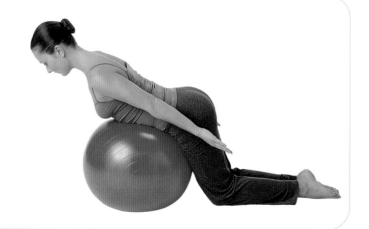

ball stretch

intermediate/advanced

For this exercise you need to choose a ball that allows you to position yourself so that your back is supported by the ball with your legs outstretched and comfortably reaching to the ground. This movement provides a stretch for the entire body, but is especially effective for stretching out your spine and releasing tension in your neck and shoulder area.

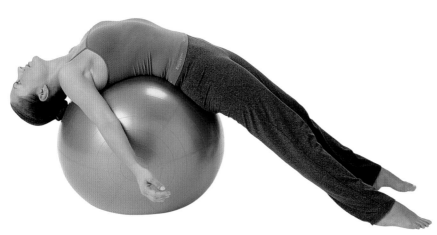

❶ Curve yourself over the exercise ball as far as you can, allowing the ball to completely support your weight. Drop your head back, but keep your neck lengthened as much as possible. Relax your arms. Extend your legs out in front of you, with your feet flat on the floor, hip-width apart. Inhale and exhale several times, allowing the ball to support you more with every exhalation and letting gravity gently stretch and release your spine and back muscles.

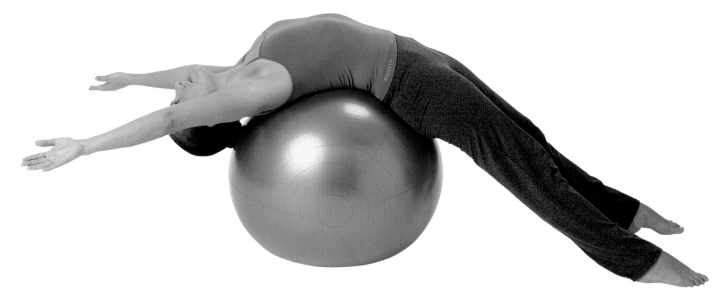

❷ Inhale, then exhale as you contract your abdominals. Continue to exhale and slowly circle your arms up toward the ceiling, then over your head and down toward the floor, lengthening them out as far as you can above your head. Inhale as you circle them down and around, back to the starting position. Keep circling your arms, using a slow, controlled movement, exhaling as you circle them up and over your head and inhaling as you bring them down and around. Do ten circles, then reverse the direction and do ten more, inhaling as you bring your arms down and around, over your head, and exhaling as you bring them up to the ceiling and down to your sides.

the hundred **with ball**

beginner/intermediate/advanced

This version of the Hundred strengthens the abdominal core and works the gluteals and the backs of the thighs. It also improves balance and stability. Choose a ball that is the correct size for you to sit with your knees bent and your feet flat on the floor in front of you.

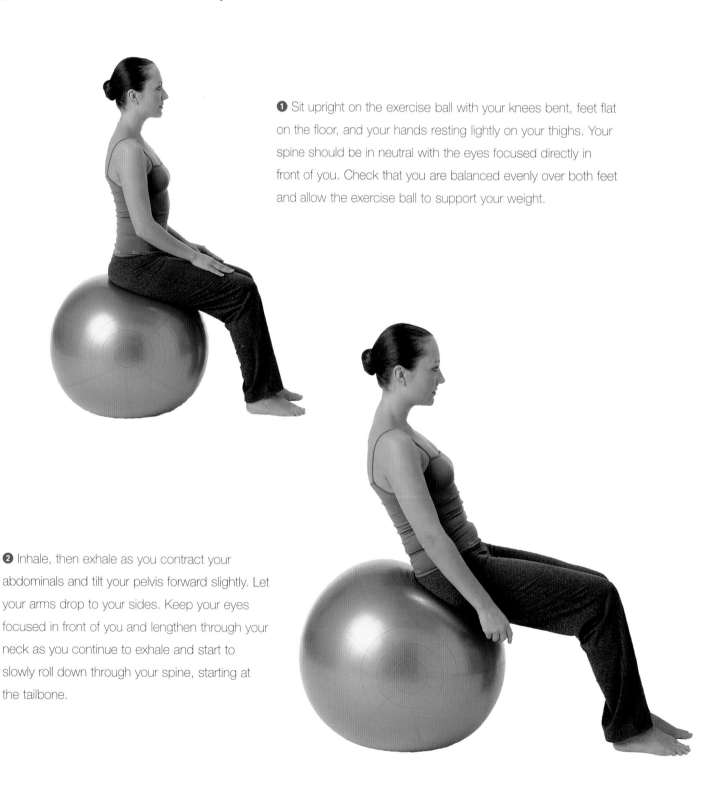

❶ Sit upright on the exercise ball with your knees bent, feet flat on the floor, and your hands resting lightly on your thighs. Your spine should be in neutral with the eyes focused directly in front of you. Check that you are balanced evenly over both feet and allow the exercise ball to support your weight.

❷ Inhale, then exhale as you contract your abdominals and tilt your pelvis forward slightly. Let your arms drop to your sides. Keep your eyes focused in front of you and lengthen through your neck as you continue to exhale and start to slowly roll down through your spine, starting at the tailbone.

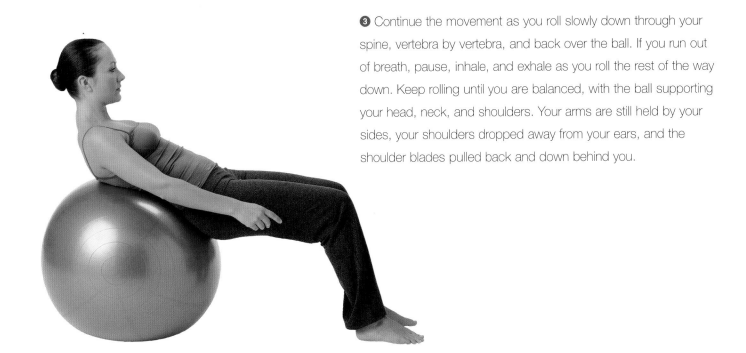

3 Continue the movement as you roll slowly down through your spine, vertebra by vertebra, and back over the ball. If you run out of breath, pause, inhale, and exhale as you roll the rest of the way down. Keep rolling until you are balanced, with the ball supporting your head, neck, and shoulders. Your arms are still held by your sides, your shoulders dropped away from your ears, and the shoulder blades pulled back and down behind you.

4 Check that your body is balanced in a parallel position, with the hips and shoulders level and your eyes looking straight up to the ceiling. Holding this position, squeeze your buttocks and and lengthen your arms, lifting and lowering them in a pulsing action, five times as you inhale and five times as you exhale, until you reach one hundred. To finish, inhale, contract your abdominals, and exhale as you roll back up to sitting using a smooth, controlled motion.

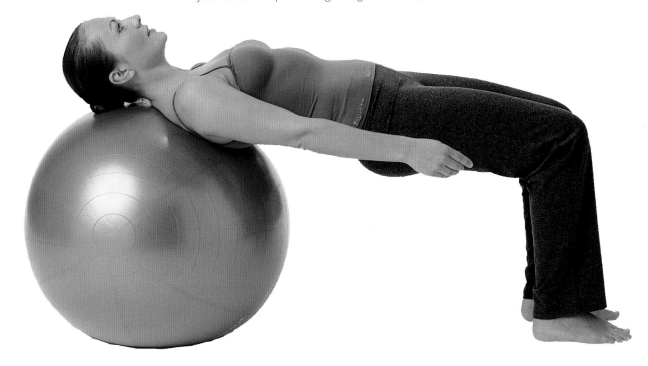

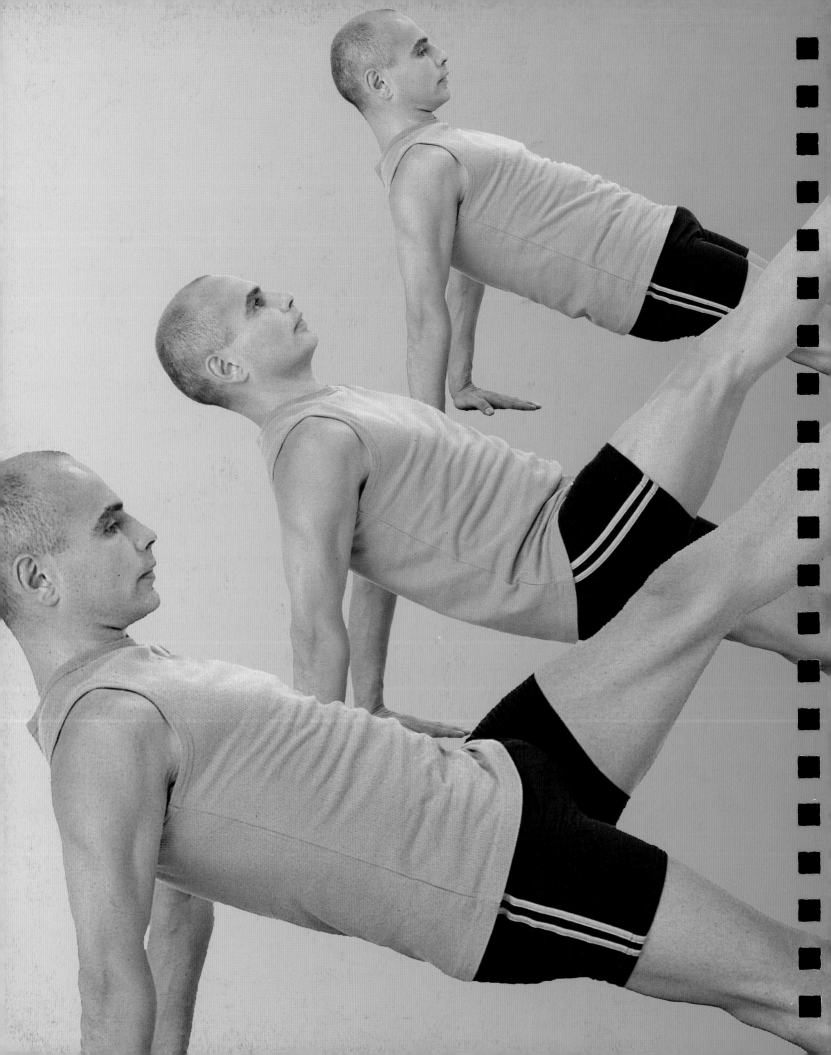

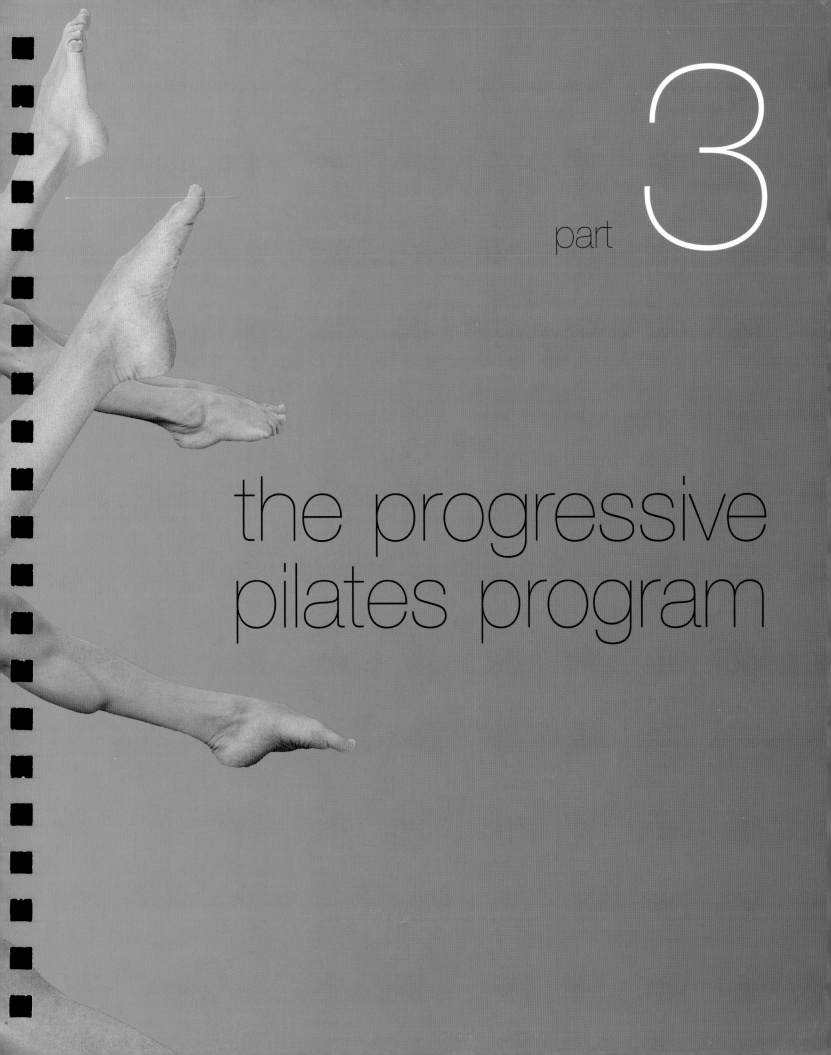

part 3

the progressive
pilates program

pilates program for beginner level

One of the advantages of the Pilates technique is that you can alter your practice routine to suit your lifestyle. To achieve any noticeable benefits, you will need to exercise for at least sixty minutes each week. How you choose to do this is up to you. You may prefer to do one sixty-minute session, two thirty-minute sessions, three twenty-minute sessions, or even daily ten-minute sessions. Experiment with the exercises and see what suits you best. The suggested routines given here for your guidance are based on twenty- to forty-minute sessions.

- Choose clothing that enables you to move freely.

- Make sure that the room is warm enough for you to feel comfortable.

- Avoid exercising if you have recently eaten a heavy meal.

- Take your time with the exercises—work at an even pace in time with your breathing.

- Always warm up and practice your breathing before you do any exercise.

- As you exercise, keep checking that your spine is in neutral with the abdominals contracted.

- If you feel any pain or discomfort, stop exercising and seek medical advice.

- Be patient with yourself—remember, the key to success is regular practice.

session 1	20	30	40	session 2	20	30	40	session 3	20	30	40	session 4	20	30	40
warm-ups	•	•	•	warm-ups	•	•	•	warm-ups	•	•	•	warm-ups	•	•	•
push-up	•	•	•	push-up	•	•	•	push-up	•	•	•	push-up	•	•	•
plank	•	•	•	swimming	•	•	•	swimming	•	•	•	chest stretch		•	•
roll up	•	•	•	plank	•	•	•	plank	•	•	•	plank	•	•	•
rolling back			•	swan dive	•	•	•	roll up	•	•	•	swimming	•	•	•
the hundred	•	•	•	roll up	•	•	•	rolling back		•	•	roll up	•	•	•
shoulder bridge	•	•	•	rolling back		•	•	the hundred	•	•	•	rolling back	•	•	•
spine stretch		•	•	the hundred	•	•	•	shoulder bridge	•	•	•	the hundred	•	•	•
the saw	•	•	•	shoulder bridge	•	•	•	the seal			•	shoulder bridge	•	•	•
the side kick			•	the side kick			•	spine stretch		•	•	one leg circles	•	•	•
one leg circles	•	•	•	one leg circles	•	•	•	the saw		•	•	one-leg stretch	•	•	•
one-leg stretch	•	•	•	one-leg stretch	•	•	•	spine twist	•	•	•	double leg kick			•
swan dive		•	•	double leg stretch	•	•	•	crab			•	double leg stretch			•
the cat			•	double leg kick			•	side bend prep			•	scissors			•
prayer	•	•	•	side bend prep		•	•	one leg circles	•	•	•	swan dive		•	•
				side bend stretch			•	one-leg stretch	•	•	•	side raises	•	•	•

pilates program for beginner level

The exercises given here are for beginner level, but could equally be performed by the more advanced student as a warm-up sequence. Detailed descriptions of the moves are given in Part 2 of this book. All movements should be

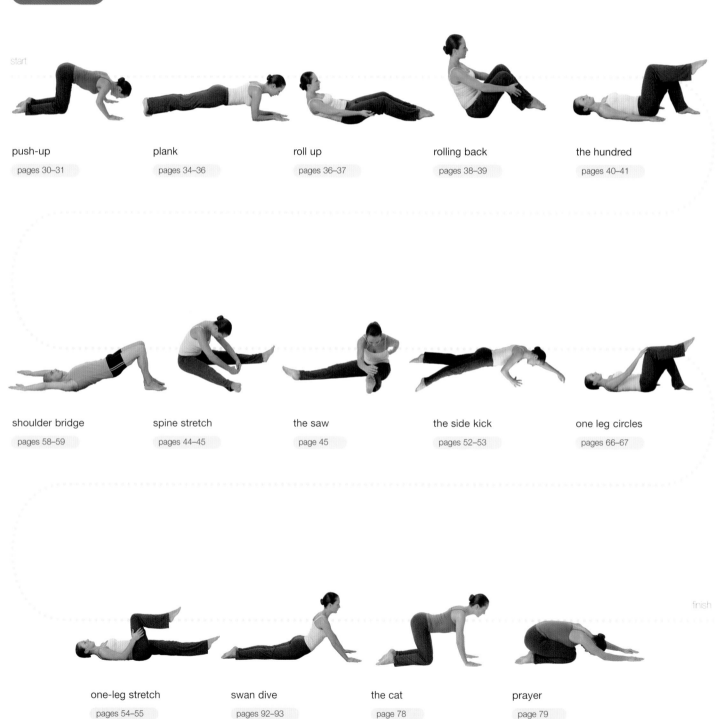

start

push-up
pages 30–31

plank
pages 34–36

roll up
pages 36–37

rolling back
pages 38–39

the hundred
pages 40–41

shoulder bridge
pages 58–59

spine stretch
pages 44–45

the saw
page 45

the side kick
pages 52–53

one leg circles
pages 66–67

one-leg stretch
pages 54–55

swan dive
pages 92–93

the cat
page 78

prayer
page 79

finish

carried out at a slow, controlled pace in time with the breathing. Focus on keeping the correct alignment of the body and supporting every move with the abdominal core, while keeping the spine in neutral.

session 2

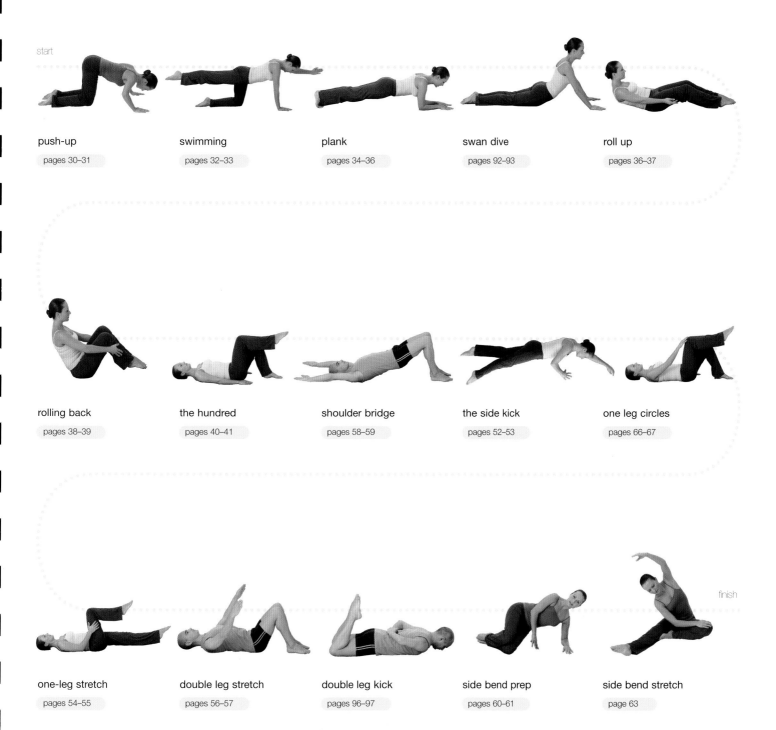

start

push-up
pages 30–31

swimming
pages 32–33

plank
pages 34–36

swan dive
pages 92–93

roll up
pages 36–37

rolling back
pages 38–39

the hundred
pages 40–41

shoulder bridge
pages 58–59

the side kick
pages 52–53

one leg circles
pages 66–67

finish

one-leg stretch
pages 54–55

double leg stretch
pages 56–57

double leg kick
pages 96–97

side bend prep
pages 60–61

side bend stretch
page 63

session 3

start

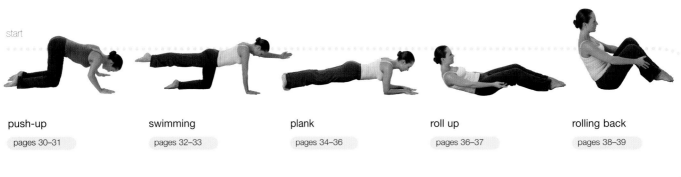

push-up
pages 30–31

swimming
pages 32–33

plank
pages 34–36

roll up
pages 36–37

rolling back
pages 38–39

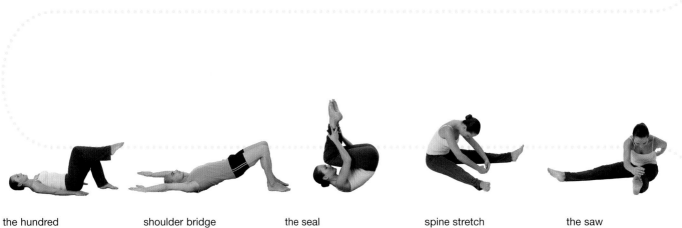

the hundred
pages 40–41

shoulder bridge
pages 58–59

the seal
page 50

spine stretch
page 44

the saw
page 45

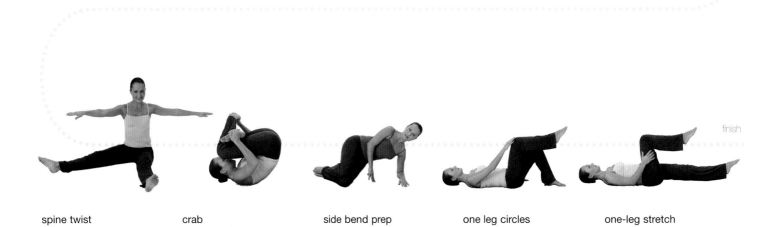

finish

spine twist
pages 46–47

crab
page 50

side bend prep
pages 60–61

one leg circles
pages 66–67

one-leg stretch
pages 54–55

session 4

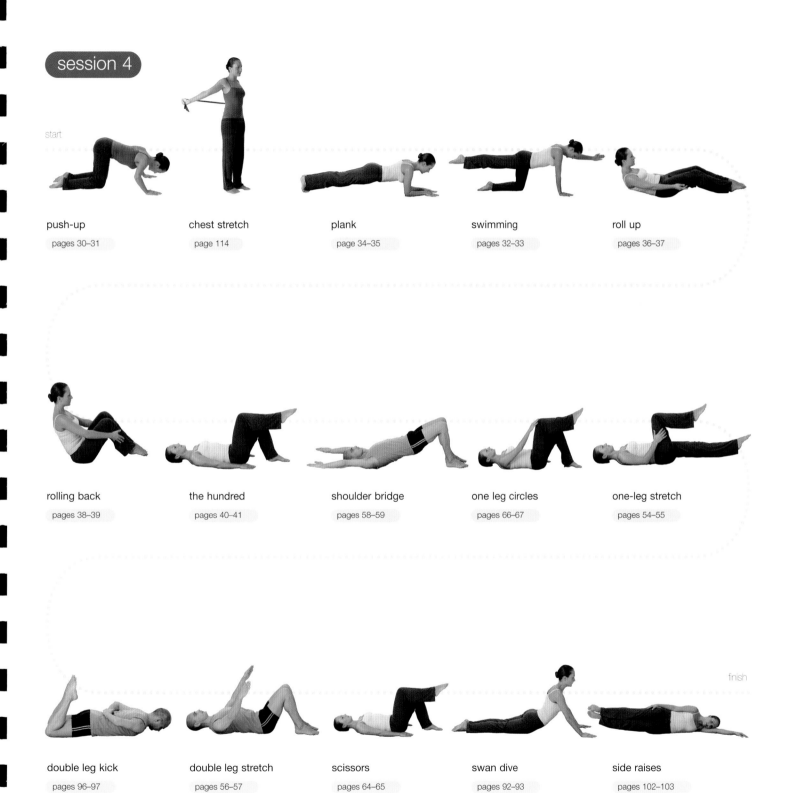

start

push-up
pages 30–31

chest stretch
page 114

plank
page 34–35

swimming
pages 32–33

roll up
pages 36–37

rolling back
pages 38–39

the hundred
pages 40–41

shoulder bridge
pages 58–59

one leg circles
pages 66–67

one-leg stretch
pages 54–55

finish

double leg kick
pages 96–97

double leg stretch
pages 56–57

scissors
pages 64–65

swan dive
pages 92–93

side raises
pages 102–103

pilates program for intermediate level

Before you attempt the intermediate level of any exercise, make sure that you have first mastered the beginner level. It is much better to work at an easier level with focus and alignment, than to struggle with an exercise that you are not yet ready for. If you are having any difficulty with a specific exercise, go back to an easier version and focus on moving more slowly and gradually increasing the number of repetitions. This will help you to increase your strength and improve your flexibility. The suggested routines given here for your guidance are based on twenty- to forty-minute sessions.

• Keep the moves slow and controlled, in rhythm with your breathing.

• If your muscles tire and you start to lose control of a move or you are no longer able to keep the abdominal contraction, reduce the number of repetitions until your stamina and strength have improved.

• Focus on keeping the spine in neutral and lengthening through the spine and the back of the neck.

• Focus on using the abdominal contraction to control each move.

• If you feel any pain or discomfort, stop exercising and seek medical advice.

• Always stretch muscles out after completing any sequence of strengthening exercises.

session 1	20	30	40	session 2	20	30	40	session 3	20	30	40	session 4	20	30	40
warm-ups	•	•	•	warm-ups	•	•	•	warm-ups	•	•	•	warm-ups	•	•	•
swimming	•	•	•	leg pull (prone)	•	•	•	swimming	•	•	•	swimming	•	•	•
plank	•	•	•	the hundred	•	•	•	the hundred	•	•	•	leg pull (prone)	•	•	•
leg pull (prone)			•	shoulder bridge	•	•	•	shoulder bridge	•	•	•	rolling back	•	•	•
roll up	•	•	•	the seal			•	side bend stretch			•	the hundred	•	•	•
rolling back			•	side kick			•	double leg stretch 2			•	shoulder bridge	•	•	•
the hundred	•	•	•	one-leg stretch	•	•	•	push-up 2	•	•	•	crab			•
shoulder bridge	•	•	•	side bend prep	•	•	•	open leg rocker			•	one leg kick	•	•	•
the seal	•	•	•	one leg circles	•	•	•	rolling into jackknife	•	•		teaser	•	•	•
spine stretch	•	•	•	side kick (kneeling)		•	•	roll over	•	•	•	neck pull prep	•	•	•
the saw	•	•	•	jackknife	•	•	•	double leg kick			•	corkscrew			•
spine twist			•	hip twist		•	•	double leg stretch 2	•	•	•	swan dive	•	•	•
one leg circles	•	•	•	neck pull prep	•	•	•	side raises	•	•	•	hip flex		•	•
one leg circles (side)		•	•	the cat			•	cancan			•	glute stretch		•	•
double leg stretch 1		•	•	prayer	•	•	•	standing pecs	•	•	•	inner thigh stretch			•
scissors	•	•	•	swan dive	•	•	•	chest stretch		•	•	hamstring	•	•	•

pilates program for intermediate level

The exercises given here are for intermediate level. Detailed descriptions of the moves are given in Part 2 of this book. As the moves become more difficult, you will need to work harder at maintaining muscle control and stability.

session 1

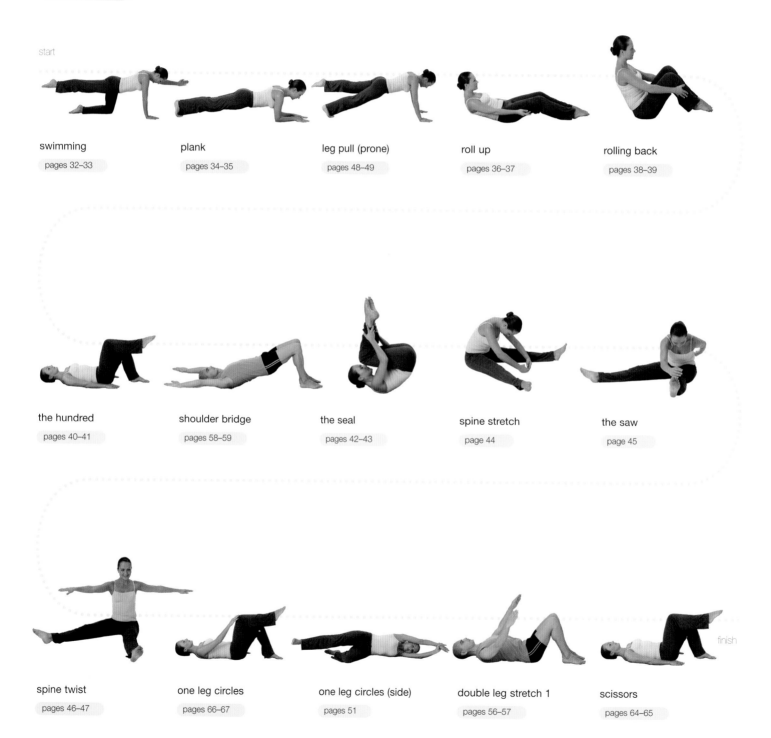

start

swimming
pages 32–33

plank
pages 34–35

leg pull (prone)
pages 48–49

roll up
pages 36–37

rolling back
pages 38–39

the hundred
pages 40–41

shoulder bridge
pages 58–59

the seal
pages 42–43

spine stretch
page 44

the saw
page 45

spine twist
pages 46–47

one leg circles
pages 66–67

one leg circles (side)
pages 51

double leg stretch 1
pages 56–57

scissors
pages 64–65

finish

Remember to move in time with the breath, keeping all your movements as smooth and fluid as possible. Avoid pushing yourself too hard—it's better to work at an easier level, keeping control, than it is to struggle beyond your ability.

session 2

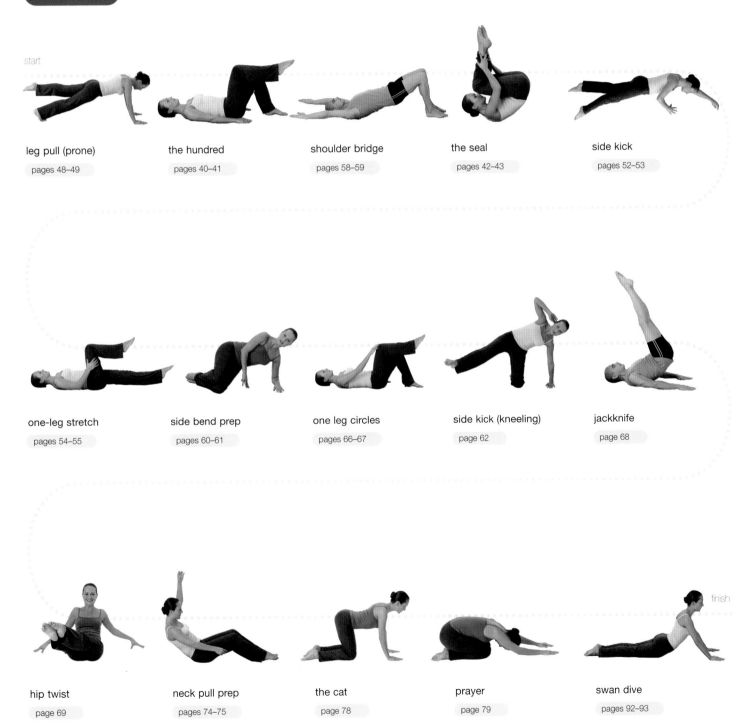

start

leg pull (prone)
pages 48–49

the hundred
pages 40–41

shoulder bridge
pages 58–59

the seal
pages 42–43

side kick
pages 52–53

one-leg stretch
pages 54–55

side bend prep
pages 60–61

one leg circles
pages 66–67

side kick (kneeling)
page 62

jackknife
page 68

hip twist
page 69

neck pull prep
pages 74–75

the cat
page 78

prayer
page 79

finish

swan dive
pages 92–93

session 3

start

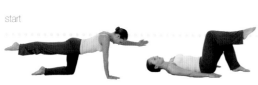

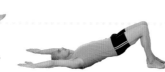

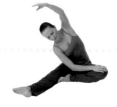

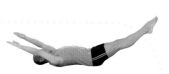

swimming

pages 32–33

the hundred

pages 40–41

shoulder bridge

pages 58–59

side bend stretch

page 53

double leg stretch 2

pages 98–99

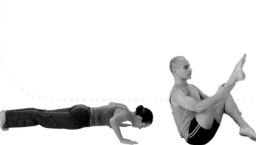

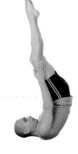

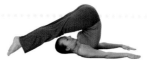

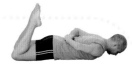

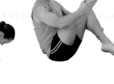

push-up 2

pages 80–81

open leg rocker

pages 82–83

rolling into jackknife

pages 88–89

roll over

pages 90–91

double leg kick

pages 96–97

finish

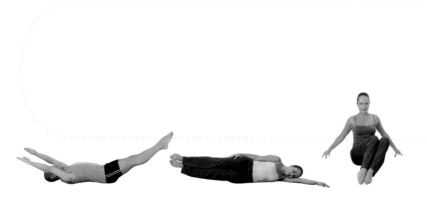

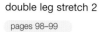

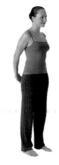

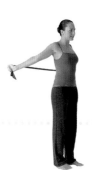

double leg stretch 2

pages 98–99

side raises

pages 102–103

cancan

pages 106–107

standing pecs

page 110

chest stretch

page 114

session 4

start

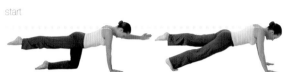

swimming	leg pull (prone)	rolling back	the hundred	shoulder bridge
pages 32–33	pages 48–49	pages 38–39	pages 40–41	pages 58–59

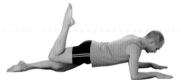
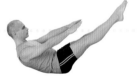
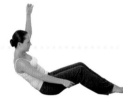
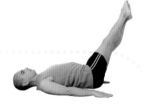

crab	one leg kick	teaser	neck pull prep	corkscrew
page 50	pages 70–71	pages 72–73	pages 74–75	pages 86–87

finish

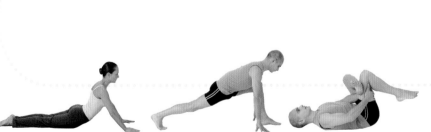
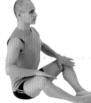
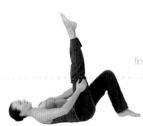

swan dive 2 & 3	hip flex	glute stretch	inner thigh stretch	hamstring
pages 100–101	pages 104–105	page 108	page 109	page 115

pilates program for advanced level

Advanced-level moves should only be attempted once you have developed a great deal of strength, flexibility, and muscle control. Avoid pushing yourself beyond your current ability—work up through the levels slowly, moving on to the next variation only when you have total confidence in your ability to do so. Pay particular attention to your abdominal core—the more difficult the move, the more you will need to use the strength and control of the abdominals to control the move and support the lower back. Keep lengthening the spine, the neck, and the limbs as you move. If you experience any pain or discomfort, stop and, if necessary, seek medical advice before continuing.

• Avoid speeding up if you find you are losing your balance—maintain a slow, controlled pace at all times.

• Always spend a few minutes warming up your muscles and practicing your breathing before embarking on your exercise routine.

• Avoid forcing any stretch—build up gradually, taking it to the point of tension and easing yourself into a final stretch.

• If you are aware that you have tension or stiffness in a particular area of your back, go slowly and don't push yourself too hard.

• If you feel any pain or discomfort, stop exercising and seek medical advice.

• Stretch out muscles at the end of any sequence of strengthening exercises.

session 1	duration (min.)			session 2	duration (min.)			session 3	duration (min.)			session 4	duration (min.)		
	20	30	40		20	30	40		20	30	40		20	30	40
warm-ups	●	●	●	warm-ups	●	●	●	warm-ups	●	●	●	warm-ups	●	●	●
swimming	●	●	●	the hundred	●	●	●	swimming	●	●	●	shoulder bridge	●	●	●
plank		●	●	shoulder bridge	●	●	●	plank	●	●	●	one leg kick	●	●	●
leg pull (prone)	●	●	●	the seal			●	the hundred			●	teaser			●
roll up		●	●	spine stretch		●	●	shoulder bridge	●	●	●	neck pull	●	●	●
rolling back	●	●	●	the saw		●	●	crab		●	●	corkscrew	●	●	●
the hundred	●	●	●	spine twist	●	●	●	one leg circles	●	●	●	side bend prone		●	●
shoulder bridge	●	●	●	side bend stretch			●	side bend prep	●	●	●	double leg kick	●	●	●
one leg circles	●	●	●	one leg circles	●	●	●	side kick (kneeling)			●	side raises	●	●	●
one leg circles (side)			●	one-leg stretch	●	●		scissors	●	●	●	hip flex	●	●	●
side kick			●	double leg stretch 2	●	●	●	neck pull	●	●	●	cancan			●
one-leg stretch	●	●		jackknife	●	●	●	the cat	●	●	●	glute stretch			●
double leg stretch 2			●	hip twist			●	prayer			●	inner thigh stretch		●	●
neck pull prep	●	●	●	neck pull prep	●	●	●	open leg rocker		●	●	hamstring	●	●	●
push-up 2	●	●	●	swan dive 2 & 3		●	●	leg pull (supine)		●	●	standing pecs	●	●	●
roll over	●	●	●	side bend prone	●	●	●	rolling into jackknife			●	chest stretch	●	●	●

pilates program for advanced level

Advanced-level moves build strength and increase flexibility in equal measure. Work your way through the variations gradually, using the easier levels to prepare you for the more difficult ones. Remember to maintain the spine in neutral

session 1

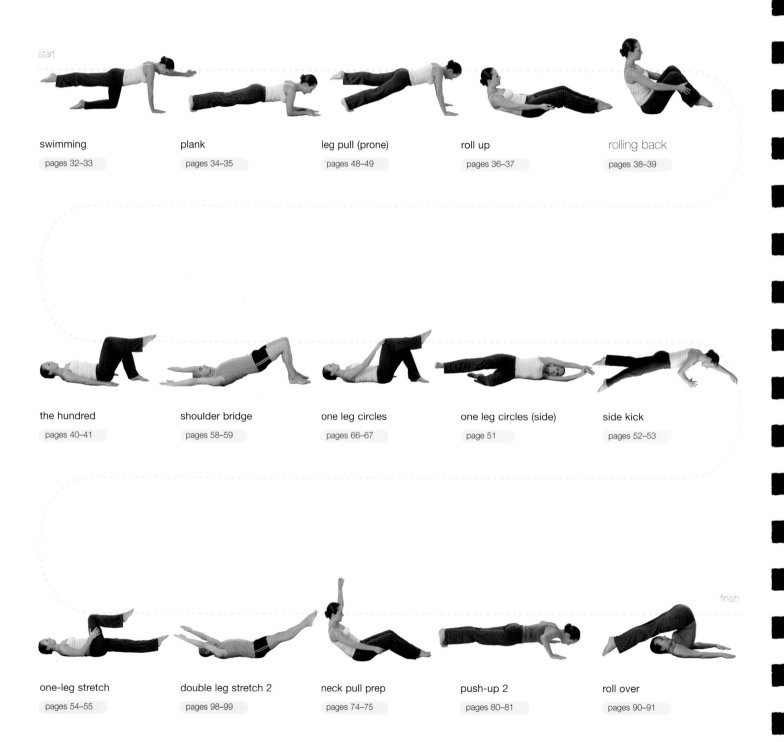

start

swimming

pages 32–33

plank

pages 34–35

leg pull (prone)

pages 48–49

roll up

pages 36–37

rolling back

pages 38–39

the hundred

pages 40–41

shoulder bridge

pages 58–59

one leg circles

pages 66–67

one leg circles (side)

page 51

side kick

pages 52–53

finish

one-leg stretch

pages 54–55

double leg stretch 2

pages 98–99

neck pull prep

pages 74–75

push-up 2

pages 80–81

roll over

pages 90–91

and contract the abdominals—avoid losing the correct body alignment in an attempt to complete a move or push it further. The suggested routines given here for your guidance are based on twenty- to forty-minute sessions.

session 2

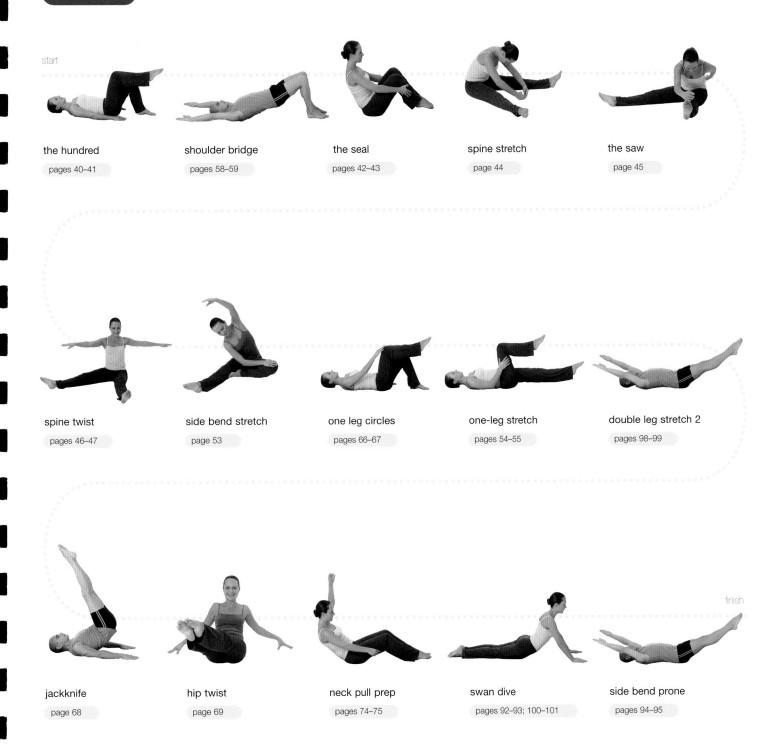

start

the hundred
pages 40–41

shoulder bridge
pages 58–59

the seal
pages 42–43

spine stretch
page 44

the saw
page 45

spine twist
pages 46–47

side bend stretch
page 53

one leg circles
pages 66–67

one-leg stretch
pages 54–55

double leg stretch 2
pages 98–99

jackknife
page 68

hip twist
page 69

neck pull prep
pages 74–75

swan dive
pages 92–93; 100–101

finish

side bend prone
pages 94–95

session 3

start

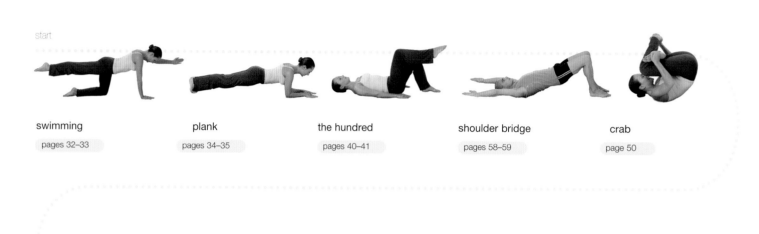

swimming

pages 32–33

plank

pages 34–35

the hundred

pages 40–41

shoulder bridge

pages 58–59

crab

page 50

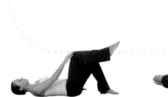

one leg circles

pages 66–67

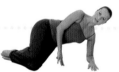

side bend prep

pages 60–61

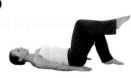

side kick (kneeling)

page 62

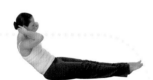

scissors

pages 64–65

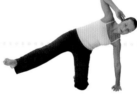

neck pull

pages 76–77

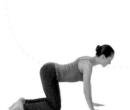

the cat

page 78

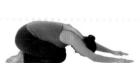

prayer

page 79

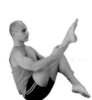

open leg rocker

pages 82–83

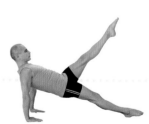

leg pull (supine)

pages 84–85

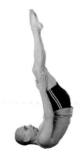

finish

rolling into jackknife

pages 88–89

session 4

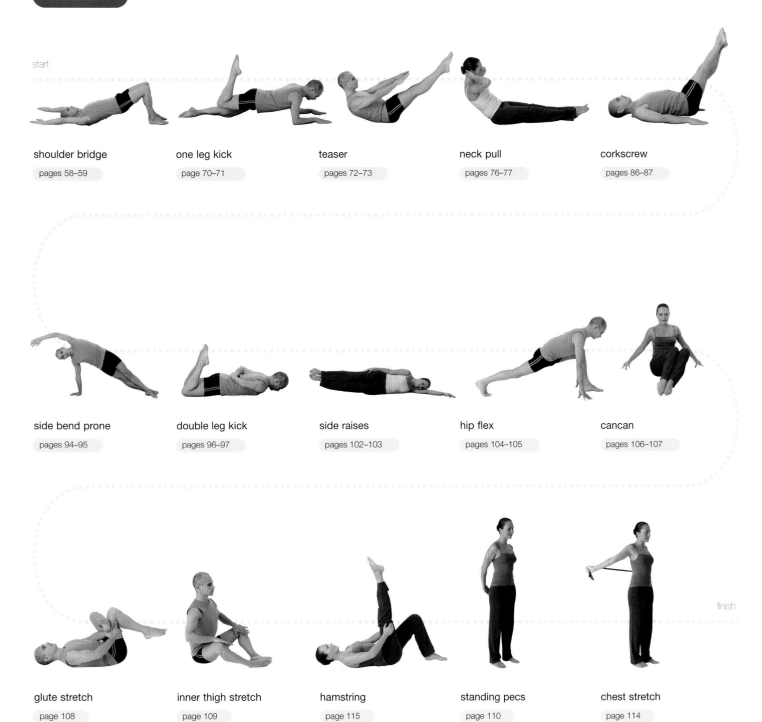

start

shoulder bridge
pages 58–59

one leg kick
page 70–71

teaser
pages 72–73

neck pull
pages 76–77

corkscrew
pages 86–87

side bend prone
pages 94–95

double leg kick
pages 96–97

side raises
pages 102–103

hip flex
pages 104–105

cancan
pages 106–107

glute stretch
page 108

inner thigh stretch
page 109

hamstring
page 115

standing pecs
page 110

chest stretch
page 114

finish

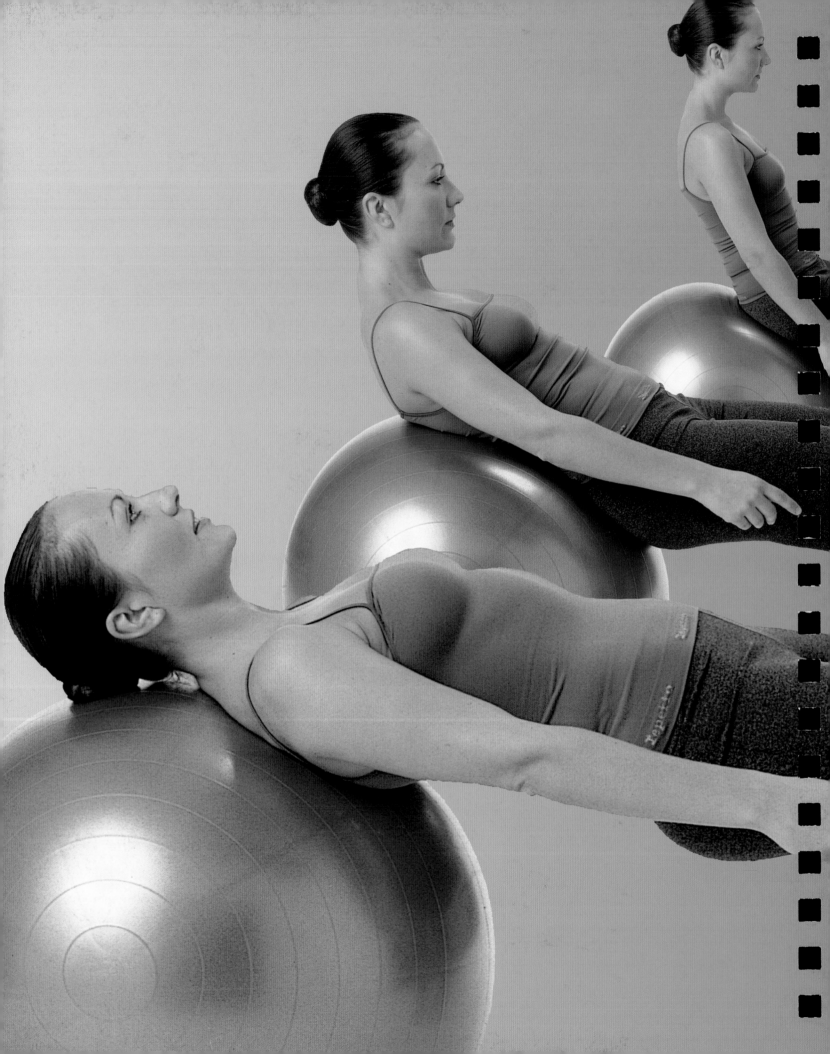

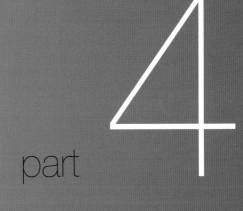

part 4

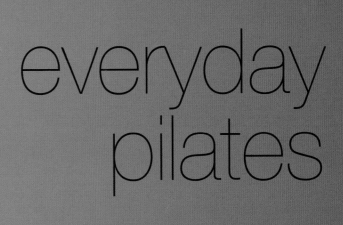

everyday
pilates

It is good to include Pilates exercises into your weekly (or even daily) schedule, but for maximum effect you need to take a close look at your daily habits and be willing to change them. Do you spend a great deal of your time slouched over a computer or slumped in front of the television? Is your lifestyle stressful and exhausting, with no time left to look after yourself properly? Do you eat regular, reasonably healthy meals, or do you tend to just grab a snack when you have a moment? The following few pages offer suggestions for short routines that you can include into your daily life, helping you to break old habits and become a new, fitter, and healthier you.

wake up routine

Taking a few minutes each morning to breathe deeply, stretch your muscles, and get your circulation going can greatly improve your energy levels and feeling of well-being. Be gentle with yourself and allow your body to wake up gradually and center itself. Choose easier levels of movements than you might use later in the day to warm and invigorate stiff, sleepy muscles.

below left: A light, nutritious breakfast is a healthy way to begin the day.
below right: Herbal teas are refreshing and a good way of avoiding caffeine.

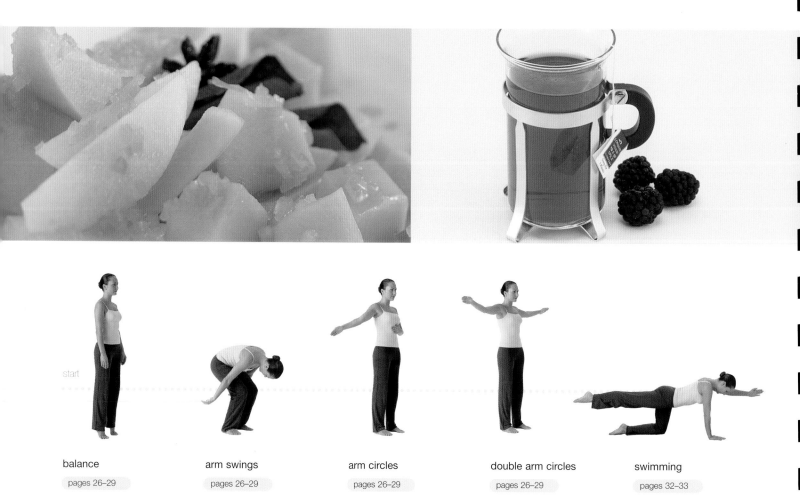

start

| balance | arm swings | arm circles | double arm circles | swimming |
| pages 26–29 | pages 26–29 | pages 26–29 | pages 26–29 | pages 32–33 |

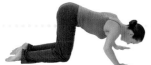

push-up 1

pages 30–31

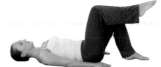

shoulder bridge

pages 58–59

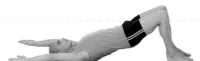

the hundred

pages 40–41

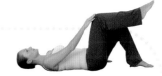

one leg circles

pages 66–67

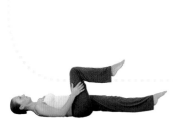

one-leg stretch

pages 54–55

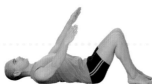

double arm stretch 1

pages 56–57

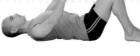

scissors

pages 64–65

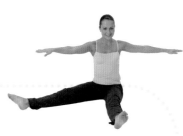

spine twist

pages 46–47

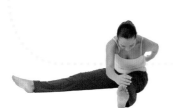

the saw

page 45

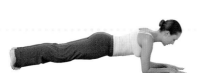

plank

pages 34–35

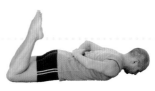

double leg kick

pages 96–97

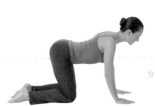

the cat

page 78

finish

energy booster

When you start to feel your energy flagging, instead of reaching for some coffee and cookies to give you a temporary lift, why not get yourself into the habit of doing a few Pilates stretches instead? Start with some breathing (pages 22–23) and warm-ups (pages 26–29), and then continue with the exercises given here. If you are pressed for time, just include as many of the moves as you have time for. But remember, however busy your schedule is, always take your time and avoid rushing the exercises—it's far better to do just two or three stretches correctly than to do more and rush them.

below left: Eat too much rich, bulky food, such as pasta with heavy sauce, and your energy levels will suffer.
below right: The refined sugar in cakes and sweets will only give you a temporary rush of energy.

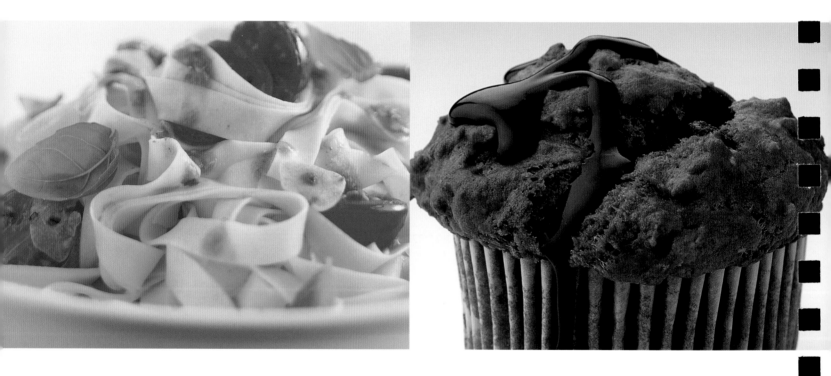

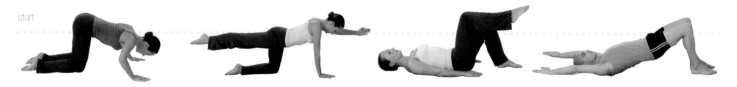

start

push-ups

pages 30–31; 80–81

swimming

pages 32–33

the hundred

pages 40–41

shoulder bridge

pages 58–59

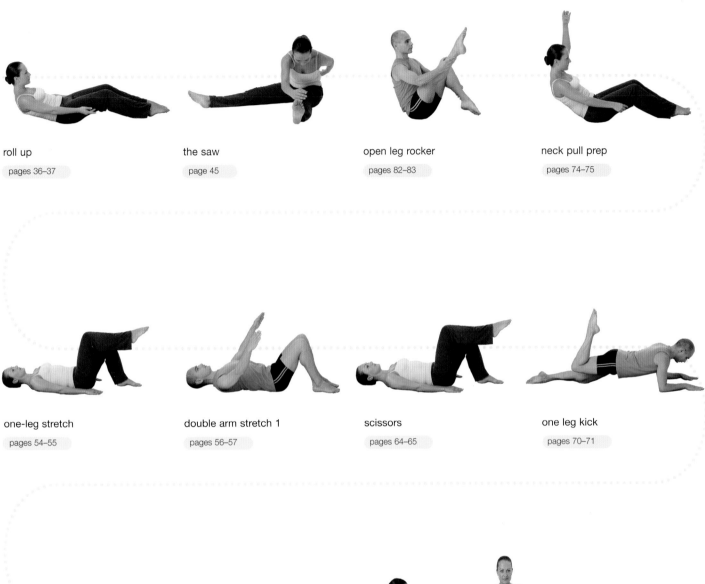

roll up

pages 36–37

the saw

page 45

open leg rocker

pages 82–83

neck pull prep

pages 74–75

one-leg stretch

pages 54–55

double arm stretch 1

pages 56–57

scissors

pages 64–65

one leg kick

pages 70–71

double leg kick

pages 96–97

swan dive

pages 92–93; 100–101

cancan

pages 106–107

finish

mental pick-me-up

For those times when you find yourself unable to think clearly, incapable of making a decision, or overwhelmed by the pressures of your responsibilities, one of the best things you can do is to take a few minutes for yourself, clear your mind, and concentrate on some Pilates techniques. These exercises will get your muscles moving and your circulation flowing. The breathing will calm you and clear your head. Even a short session of exercises will allow your to return to your activities and responsibilities feeling invigorated, refreshed, and revitalized.

below left: A few moments of creative visualization can be a big help when you're in need of mental relaxation.

below right: With their high levels of potassium, bananas are good brain food.

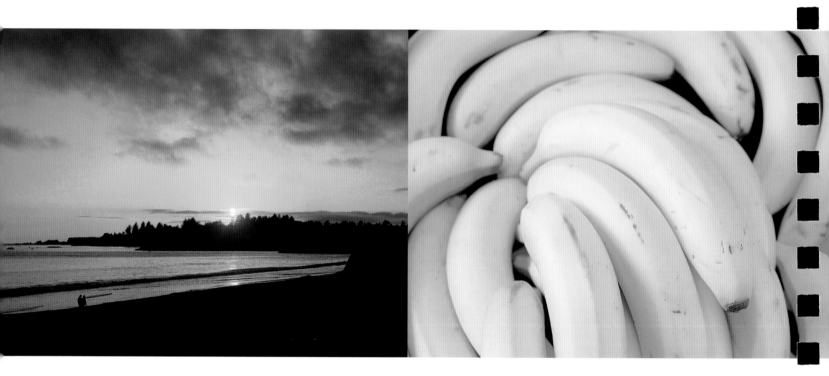

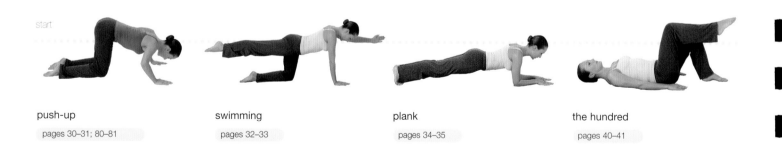

start

push-up

pages 30–31; 80–81

swimming

pages 32–33

plank

pages 34–35

the hundred

pages 40–41

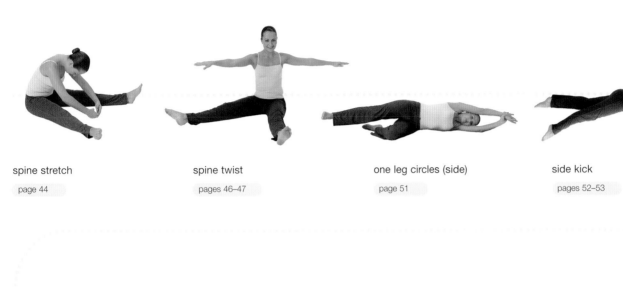

spine stretch

page 44

spine twist

pages 46–47

one leg circles (side)

page 51

side kick

pages 52–53

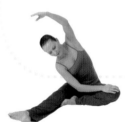 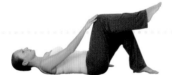 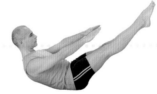 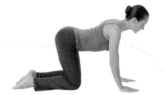

side bend stretch

page 63

one leg circles

pages 66–67

teaser

pages 72–73

the cat

page 78

finish

 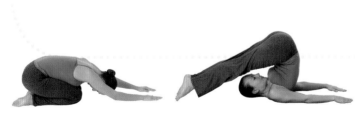 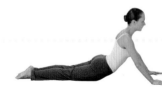 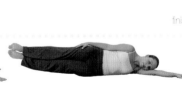

prayer

page 79

roll over

pages 90–91

swan dive

pages 92–93; 100–101

side raises

pages 102–103

de-stress and rebalance

The way we live our lives is reflected in our bodies, and living under constant stress will have an effect upon our well-being. If we are unable to reduce the amount of pressure we have to deal with on a day-to-day basis, then we need to learn to function more efficiently so that it has less of an undermining effect upon our mental, emotional, and physical states. Taking time out, getting sufficient rest, and eating a healthy diet are essential factors, while making sure that our bodies are as strong, flexible, and resilient as possible will increase our ability to cope with life's challenges, and allow us to find the resources within ourselves to take charge of events and manage our lives more constructively. Even a regular short session of Pilates will leave us feeling rebalanced in mind and body, able to cope with pressures that previously overwhelmed us. Spend a minute or two practicing Pilates breathing and finding your neutral position, then try as many of the following exercises as you have time for.

below left: Lavender can be a good treatment for insomnia and restlessness, and can help you relax.

below right: Visualization of calming scenes or images is an important part of meditation and relaxation.

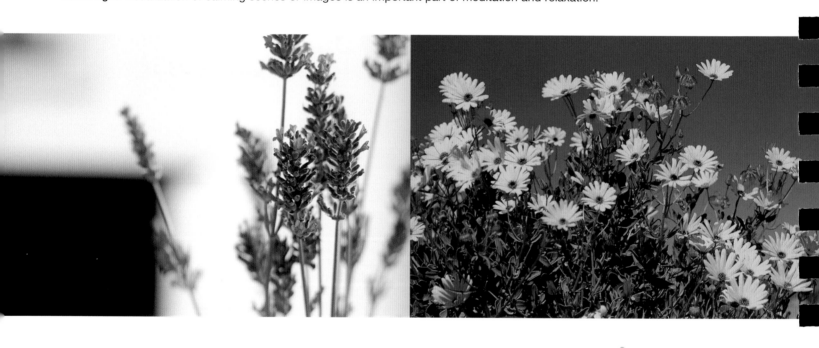

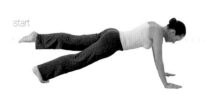

start

leg pull (prone)

pages 48–49

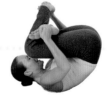

crab

page 50

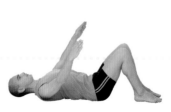

double arm stretch 1

pages 56–57

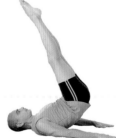

jackknife

page 68

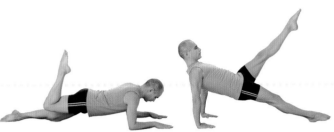

one leg kick

pages 70–71

leg pull (supine)

pages 84–85

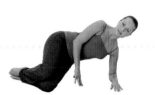

side bend prep

pages 60–61

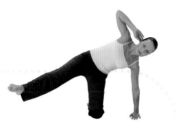

side kick (kneeling)

page 62

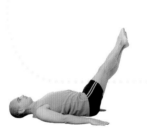

corkscrew

pages 86–87

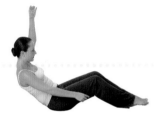

neck pull prep

pages 74–75

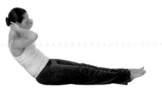

neck pull prone

pages 76–77

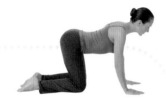

the cat

page 78

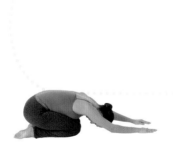

prayer

page 79

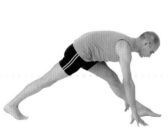

hip flex

pages 104–105

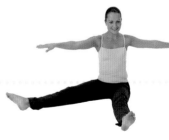

spine twist

pages 46–47

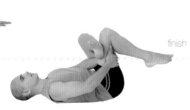
finish

glute stretch

page 108

stamina workout

Pilates is not a replacement for other forms of exercise and learning the Pilates technique does not mean that you will have to give up any other form of fitness training. Indeed, Pilates is an ideal form of exercise to combine with other, more aerobic programs as it strengthens the body, improves muscle tone and control, stimulates the circulation, increases flexibility, improves balance, and corrects postural problems. However, as you develop, you will find that Pilates can provide an extremely demanding, satisfying body workout, increasing stamina, building strength, and improving flexibility. Take a few minutes to prepare and warm up (pages 22–23 and 26–29), then follow the sequence of exercises given here. Avoid pushing yourself too far. It is better to work at an easier level for a while longer, adding more repetitions and slowing down the move to increase the level of difficulty, to build up your strength and muscle control. If you feel any pain or discomfort, stop immediately and seek medical advice before continuing.

below left: Eating fresh fruit or vegetables before an activity is a great way of maintaining your stamina.

below right: Rest and relaxation are as important as regular exercise for a balanced lifestyle.

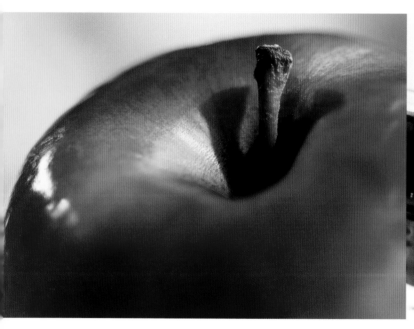
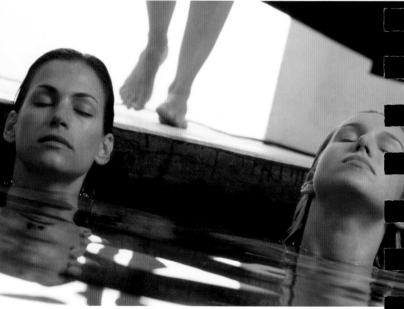

start

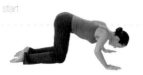
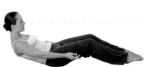
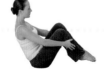
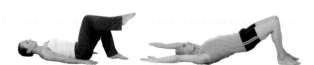

push-up	roll up	rolling back	the hundred	shoulder bridge
pages 30–31; 80–81	pages 36–37	pages 38–39	pages 40–41	pages 58–59

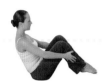

the seal

pages 42–43

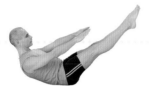

teaser

pages 72–73

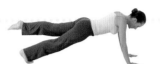

leg pull (prone)

pages 48–49

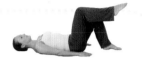

scissors

pages 64–65

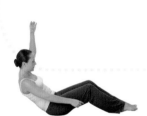

neck pull prep

pages 74–75

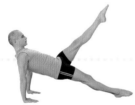

leg pull (supine)

pages 84–85

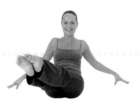

hip twist

page 69

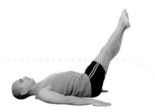

corkscrew

pages 86–87

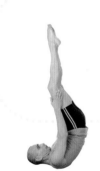

rolling into jackknife

pages 88–89

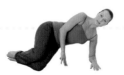

side bend prone

pages 94–95

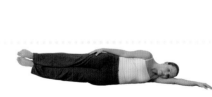

side raises

pages 102–103

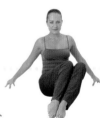

cancan

pages 106–107

finish

evening wind down

A slow, relaxing session of Pilates can be the perfect antidote to a busy day and will calm your body, clear your mind, and help you relax and unwind. Begin your evening routine with some warm-up exercises (see pages 26–29), then lie on your back for a few exercises, with your knees bent up to the ceiling, your spine in neutral, and eyes closed, and take several deep breaths. Once you have finished the sequence of exercises, return to this position once more for a few minutes, making sure your back is in neutral with your spine and neck lengthened, and focus on your breathing—imagine your back melting into the floor and your chest softening and relaxing. You may find it more comfortable to place a small pillow or a folded towel under your head. Keep your knees pointing straight up to the ceiling and your arms relaxed by your sides.

below left: It's best to keep your last meal of the day light, as heavy evening meals can cause indigestion and keep you from sleeping soundly.

below right: Pampering yourself at the end of the day can help you relax and unwind.

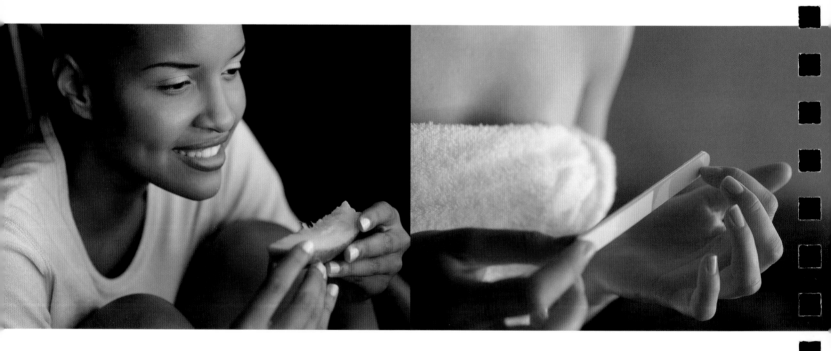

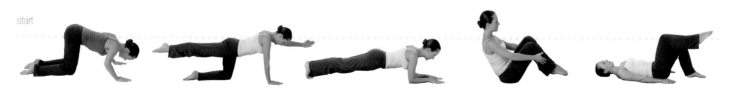

start

push-up	swimming	plank	rolling back	the hundred
pages 30–31; 80–81	pages 32–33	pages 34–35	pages 38–39	pages 40–41

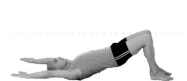

shoulder bridge

pages 58–59

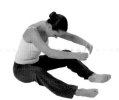

spine stretch

page 44

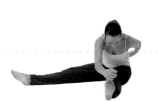

the saw

page 45

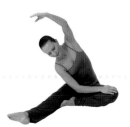

side bend stretch

page 63

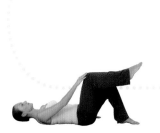

one leg circles

pages 66–67

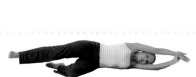

one leg circles (side)

page 51

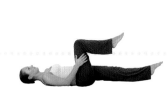

one-leg stretch

pages 54–55

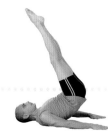

jackknife

page 68

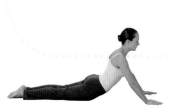

swan dive

pages 92–93; 100–101

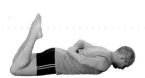

double leg kick

pages 96–97

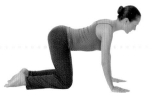

the cat

page 78

finish

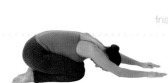

prayer

page 79

bedtime relaxation

Finishing the day with a few minutes of slow, gentle Pilates stretches can help ensure a good night's sleep. Make sure the room is sufficiently warm, light some candles, and put on some soothing music. Start by lying on your back with your knees bent and pointing straight up to the ceiling, and your feet placed flat on the floor in parallel, hip-width apart, and your arms relaxed by your sides. Take a few deep breaths and let any stressful thoughts just melt away. Take a few minutes to take your attention down through your body, starting with your head and slowly working down to your feet. Notice any places that you are holding any tension and imagine breathing into that place, dissolving any feeling of tightness or stiffness. When you have finished your stretches, repeat this position for a few more minutes, concentrating on taking slow, deep breaths.

below left: Incense is a traditional form of aromatherapy and can aid relaxation.

below right: A firm mattress is essential for a good night's rest.

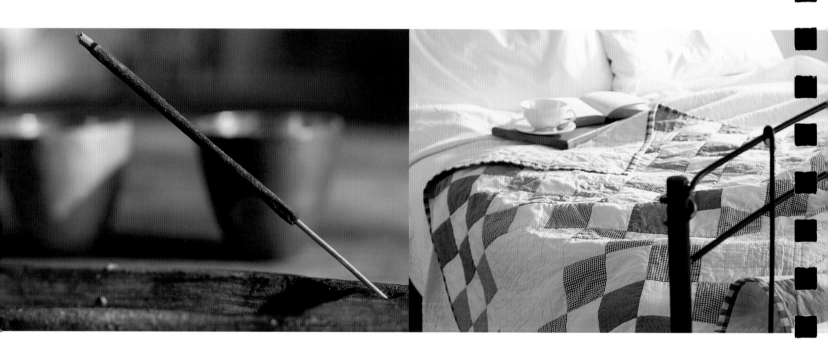

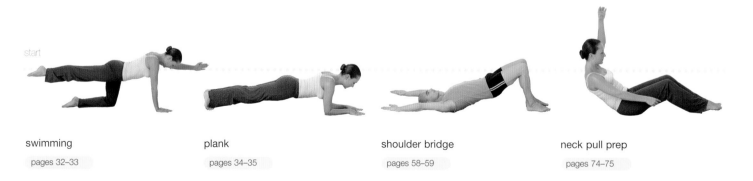

start

swimming

pages 32–33

plank

pages 34–35

shoulder bridge

pages 58–59

neck pull prep

pages 74–75

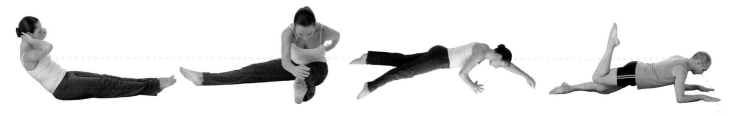

neck pull prone

pages 76–77

the saw

page 45

side kick

pages 52–53

one-leg stretch

pages 54–55

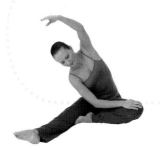

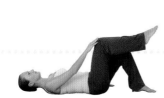

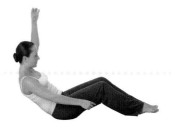

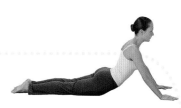

side bend stretch

page 63

one leg circles

pages 66–67

neck pull prep

pages 74–75

swan dive

pages 92–93; 100–101

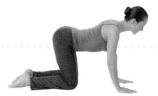

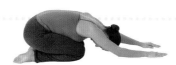

finish

the cat

page 78

prayer

page 79

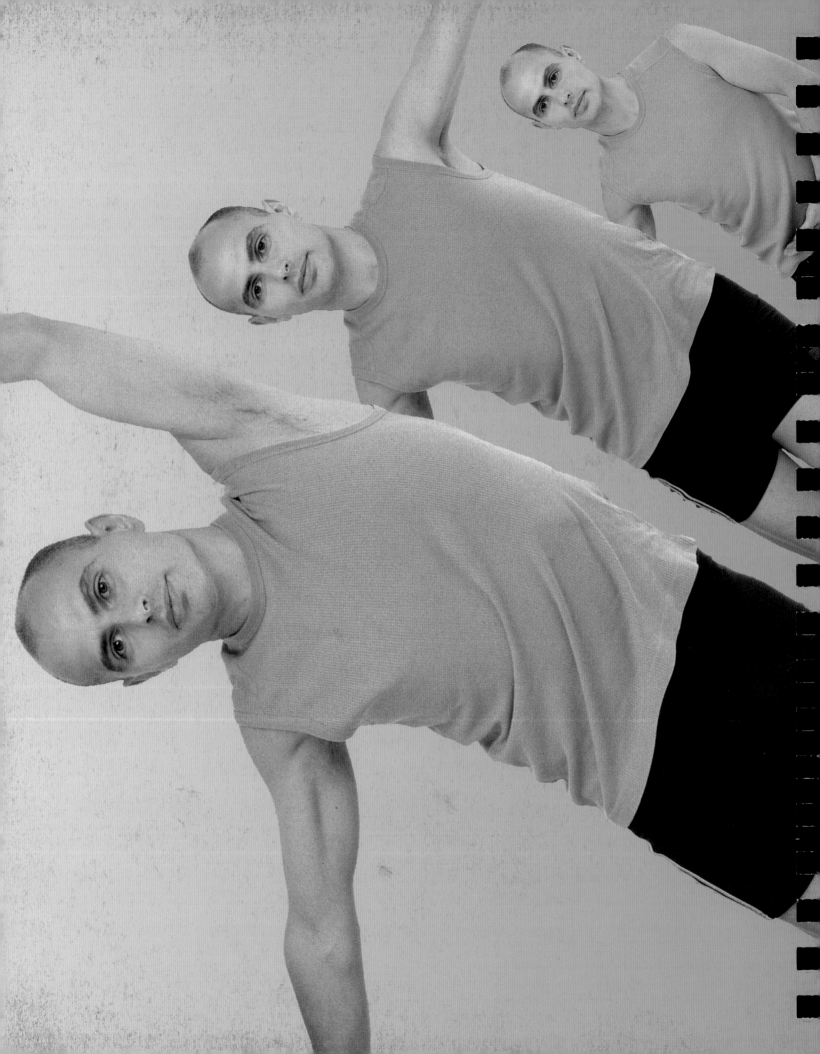

healing pilates

standing activities

If your daily activities require that you spend a lot of your time on your feet, you may be prone to aching legs and back, stiffness, sore feet, or even circulation problems. The following exercises are an excellent addition to your usual routine and will help to improve posture and balance, reduce tension, and relieve stiffness and discomfort. Regular practice will help prevent future problems from occurring.

below left: A good foot massage can help you forget the pain and strain of standing on your feet all day.

below right: Oily fish are good for the circulation, which can become sluggish if you're on your feet a lot.

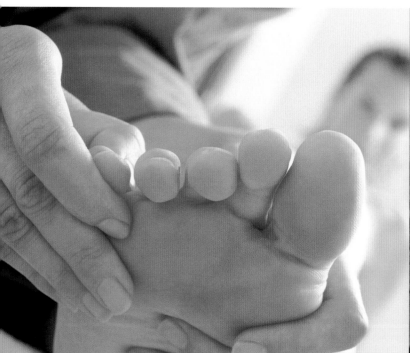
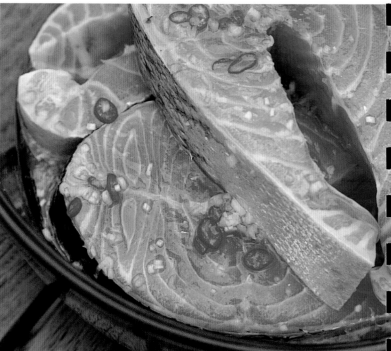

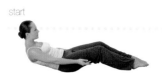

roll up

pages 36–37

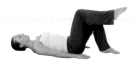

the hundred

pages 40–41

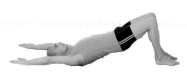

shoulder bridge

pages 58–59

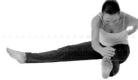

the saw

page 45

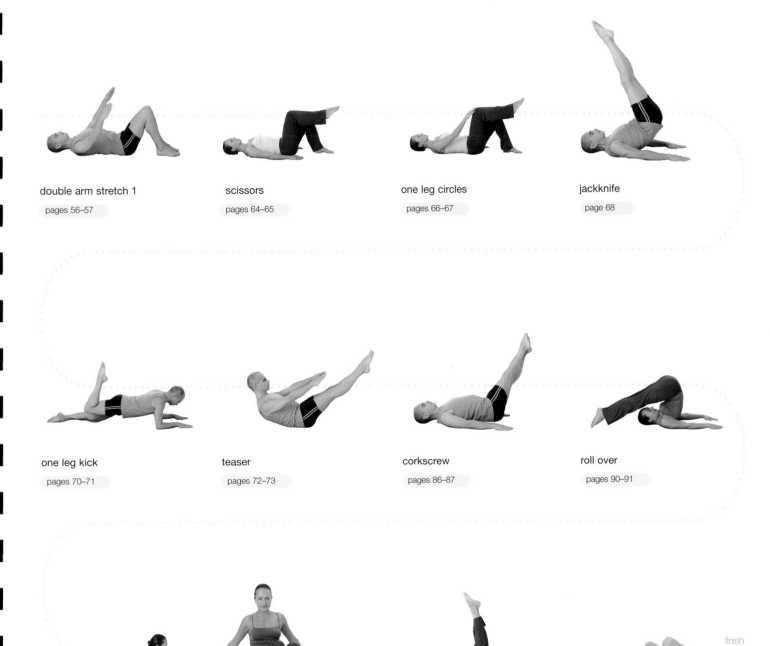

double arm stretch 1

pages 56–57

scissors

pages 64–65

one leg circles

pages 66–67

jackknife

page 68

one leg kick

pages 70–71

teaser

pages 72–73

corkscrew

pages 86–87

roll over

pages 90–91

swan dive

pages 92–93; 100–101

cancan

pages 106–107

hamstring

page 115

glute stretch

page 108

finish

sitting activities

If your daily activities require that you spend much of your day sitting, either at a desk or behind the wheel of a car, for example, you will benefit from including exercises in your regular routine to help counteract any detrimental effects that this might cause. Sitting without movement for any length of time can cause stiffness in the lower back, tightness in the hips, and discomfort in the legs. If you work at a computer or spend much time driving, you may develop tension in your neck and shoulders. Try to take a few minutes in your day to stretch out and rebalance your body.

below left: Avoid heavy lunchtime meals, especially if you have a sedentary job, as you're doing little to burn up energy.

below right: Swimming is a good antidote to sitting at your desk or being stuck behind the wheel of a car.

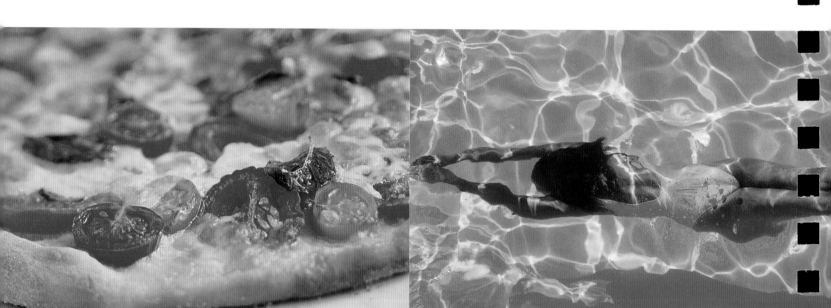

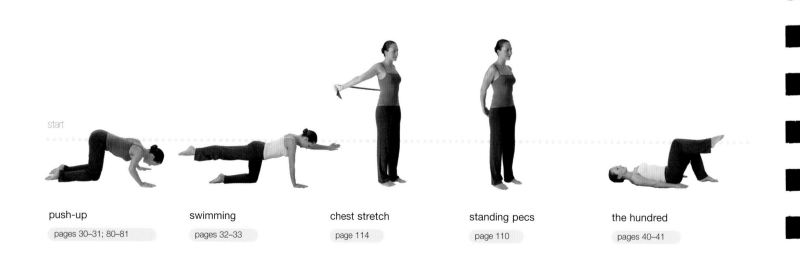

start

push-up	swimming	chest stretch	standing pecs	the hundred
pages 30–31; 80–81	pages 32–33	page 114	page 110	pages 40–41

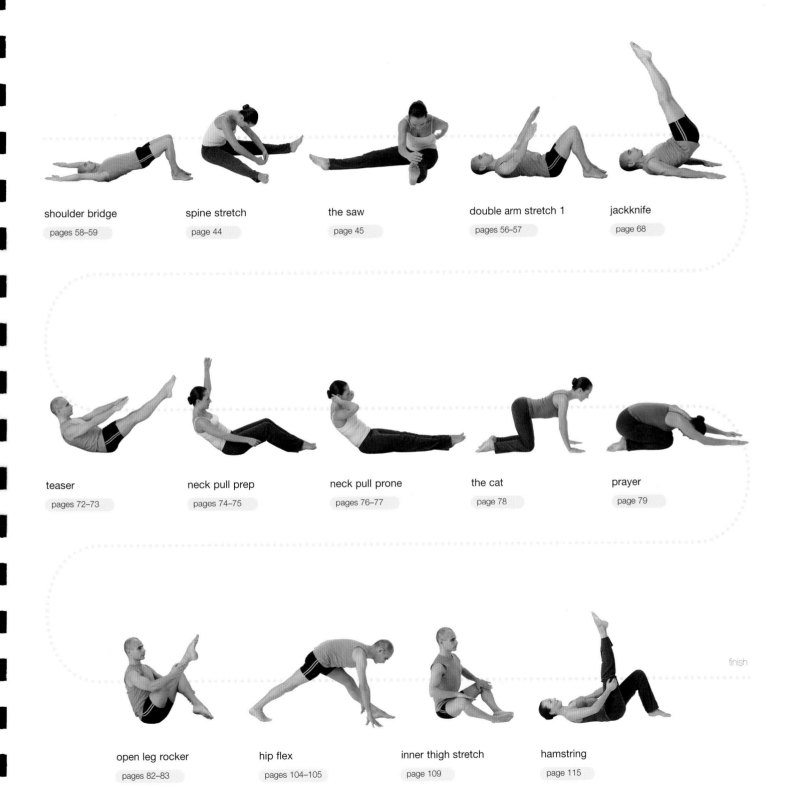

shoulder bridge

pages 58–59

spine stretch

page 44

the saw

page 45

double arm stretch 1

pages 56–57

jackknife

page 68

teaser

pages 72–73

neck pull prep

pages 74–75

neck pull prone

pages 76–77

the cat

page 78

prayer

page 79

open leg rocker

pages 82–83

hip flex

pages 104–105

inner thigh stretch

page 109

hamstring

page 115

finish

pilates for headaches

Headaches are frequently caused by muscle tension in the neck and shoulders, bad posture, poor circulation, stress, and exhaustion. Regularly stretching the body with Pilates exercises can help improve your posture, release tension and stiffness, and relieve stress, relaxing your mind and body, reducing aches and pains, and helping to prevent them from occurring in the future. Over time it will also improve your body awareness, allowing you to notice the early warning signs of headaches or other aches and pains and take preventive action.

below left: Food allergies are a common cause of headaches, and the tannins in alcohol are often a prime culprit.

below right: A massage to the face, head, and neck can help relieve headaches.

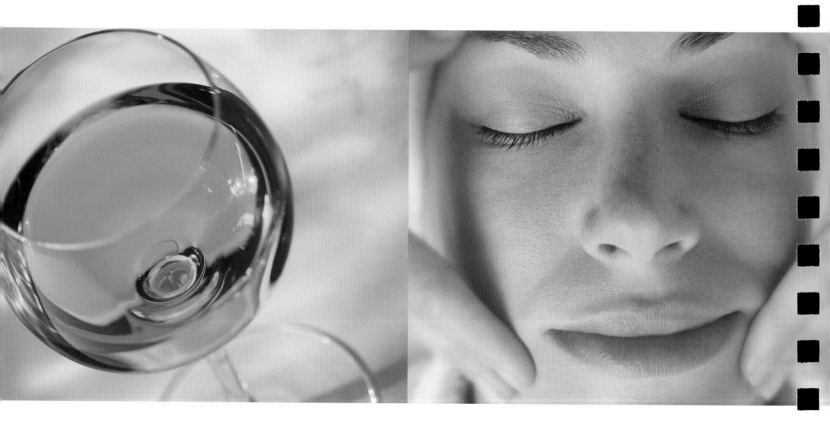

start

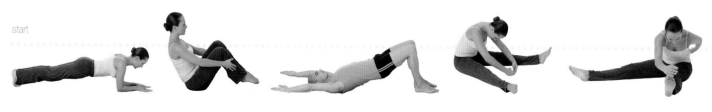

plank	rolling back	shoulder bridge	spine stretch	the saw
pages 34–35	pages 38–39	pages 58–59	page 44	page 45

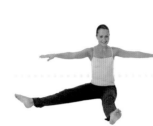

spine twist

pages 46–47

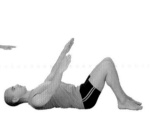

double arm stretch 1

pages 56–57

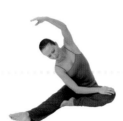

side bend stretch

page 63

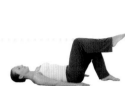

scissors

pages 64–65

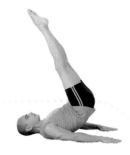

jackknife

page 68

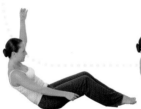

neck pull prep

pages 74–75

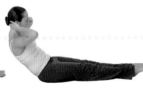

neck pull prone

pages 76–77

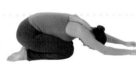

prayer

page 79

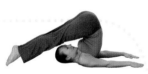

open leg rocker

pages 82–83

roll over

pages 90–91

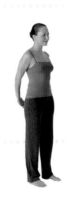

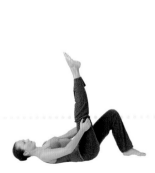

hamstring

page 115

standing pecs

page 110

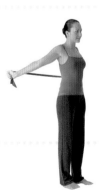

chest stretch

page 114

finish

pilates for back problems

If you suffer from any back or neck problems, it is essential that you seek medical advice before embarking on any system of exercise—there are some conditions for which exercise is not recommended. However, most cases of back pain are caused by bad posture, tension in the neck and shoulders, or even stress, and can be greatly improved by appropriate, regular exercise. The Pilates technique will help to eliminate bad postural habits while strengthening the muscles, increasing muscle control, and improving balance and flexibility. If you experience any pain or discomfort while stretching, then stop immediately and refer to your medical practitioner.

below left: The buoyancy and support provided by water makes swimming a good exercise for people with back problems.

below right: A good massage can help a lot with back problems—but consult a doctor first.

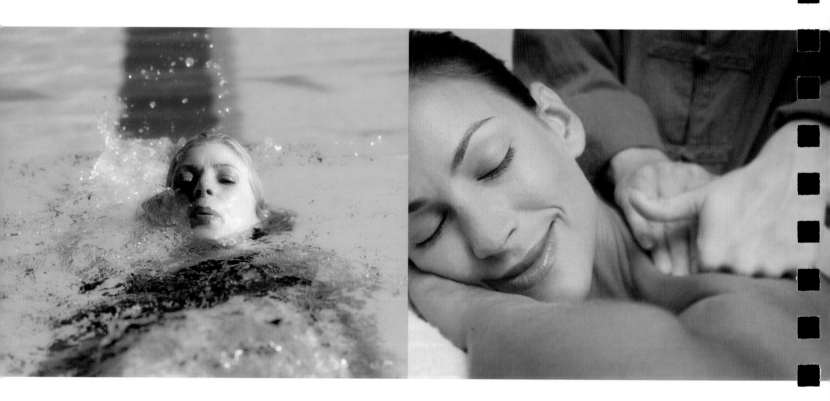

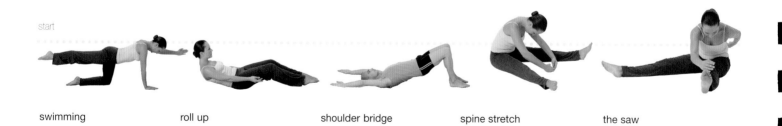

start

swimming	roll up	shoulder bridge	spine stretch	the saw
pages 32–33	pages 36–37	pages 58–59	page 44	page 45

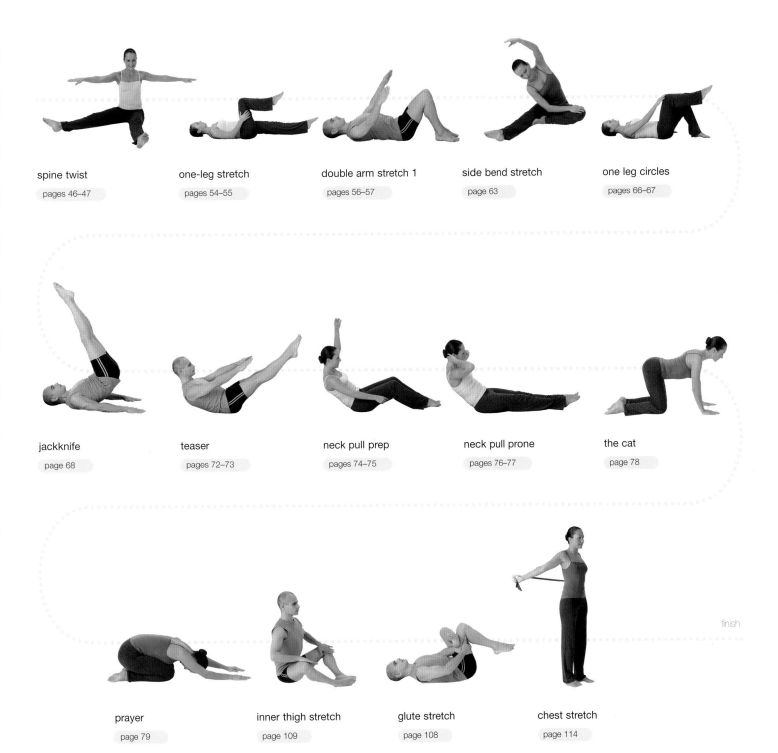

spine twist

pages 46–47

one-leg stretch

pages 54–55

double arm stretch 1

pages 56–57

side bend stretch

page 63

one leg circles

pages 66–67

jackknife

page 68

teaser

pages 72–73

neck pull prep

pages 74–75

neck pull prone

pages 76–77

the cat

page 78

prayer

page 79

inner thigh stretch

page 109

glute stretch

page 108

chest stretch

page 114

finish

pilates to boost the immune system

Exercise is an excellent way to boost the immune system and Pilates is no exception. Regular practice of Pilates strengthens the body and improves breathing and circulation, ensuring that your immune system is in top condition.

below left: Oranges are a good source of vitamin C, which is said to boost the immune system.

below right: Regular exercise helps keep the body fit and healthy, and stimulates your immune system.

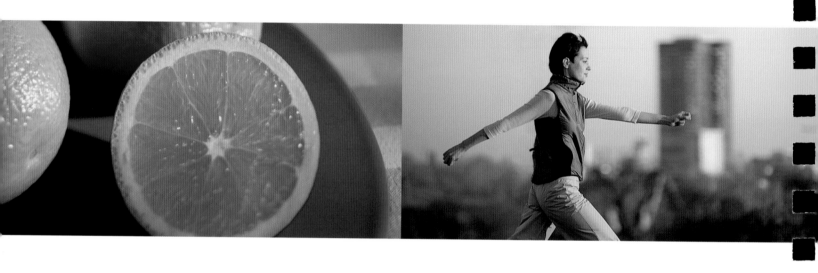

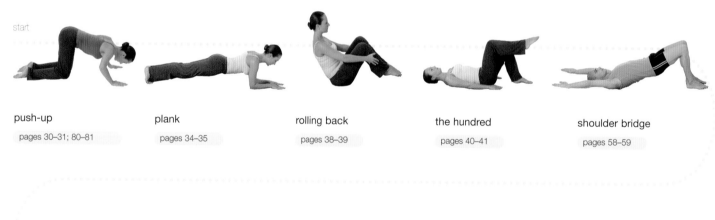

start

push-up

pages 30–31; 80–81

plank

pages 34–35

rolling back

pages 38–39

the hundred

pages 40–41

shoulder bridge

pages 58–59

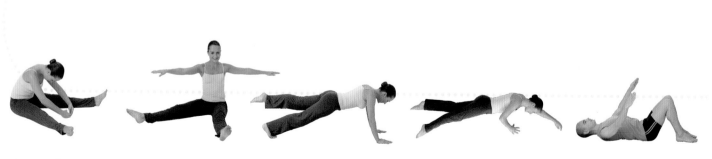

spine stretch

page 44

spine twist

pages 46–47

leg pull (prone)

pages 48–49

side kick

pages 52–53

double arm stretch 1

pages 56–57

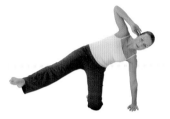

side kick (kneeling)

page 62

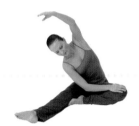

side bend stretch

page 63

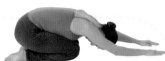

neck pull prep or neck pull prone

pages 74–77

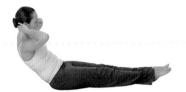

prayer

page 79

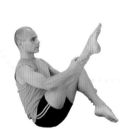

open leg rocker

pages 82–83

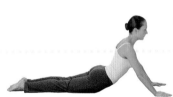

swan dive

pages 92–93; 100–101

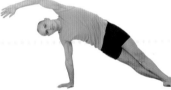

side bend prone

pages 94–95

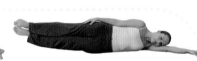

side raises

pages 102–103

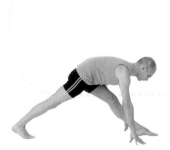

hip flex

pages 104–105

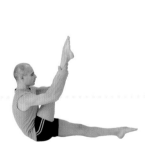

climb tree

page 113

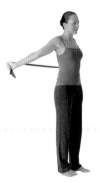

chest stretch

page 114

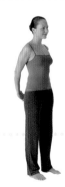

finish

standing pecs

page 110

pilates for flying

For many of us, flying can be a very stressful experience, even before we actually take off. Preparing, packing, carrying heavy suitcases, and the stress of rushing to get everything organized before we go away can all take their toll on our bodies. Once in the air, growing fatigue and having to sit in one position for several hours add to our general discomfort and increasing tension and stiffness. Nowadays, with fears of deep vein thrombosis and a growing awareness of the importance of maintaining our well-being, we are encouraged to get out of our seats every so often and stretch out our muscles when we fly. Performing some Pilates exercises prior to traveling and trying some gentle stretches in the air will help you to overcome the stresses and strains of flying.

below left: Avoid drinking alcohol on long flights, as it will add to the dehydration—drink plenty of water.

below right: Use a pillow to give your head a comfortable resting position and support your neck.

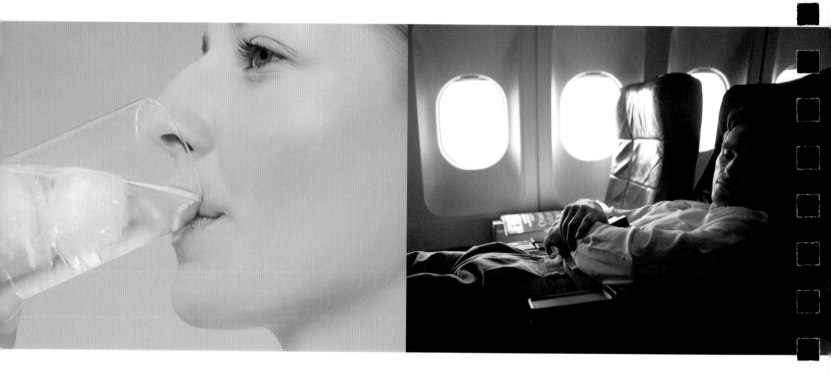

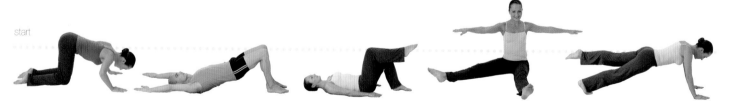

start

push-up	shoulder bridge	the hundred	spine twist	leg pull (prone)
pages 30–31; 80–81	pages 58–59	pages 40–41	pages 46–47	pages 48–49

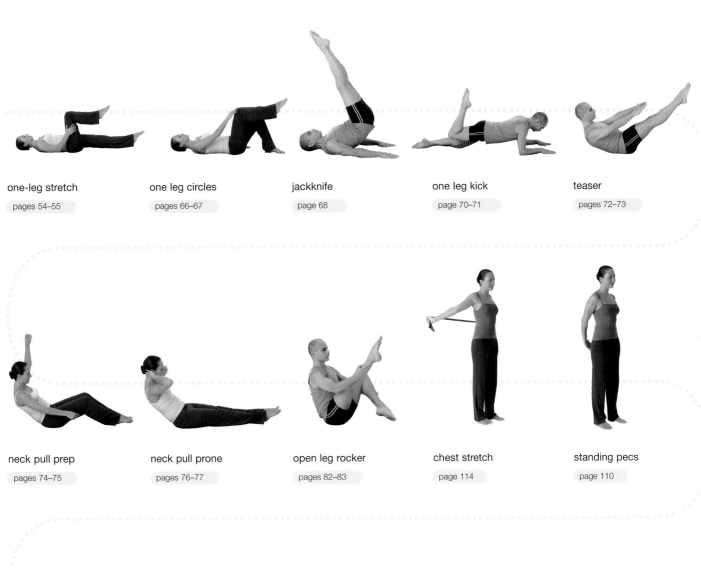

one-leg stretch
pages 54–55

one leg circles
pages 66–67

jackknife
page 68

one leg kick
page 70–71

teaser
pages 72–73

neck pull prep
pages 74–75

neck pull prone
pages 76–77

open leg rocker
pages 82–83

chest stretch
page 114

standing pecs
page 110

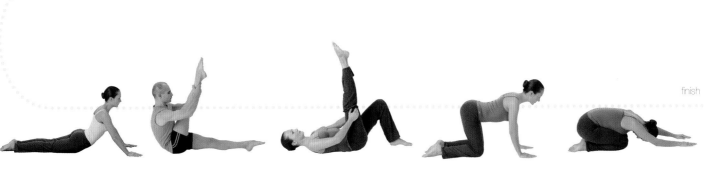

finish

swan dive
pages 92–93; 100–101

climb tree
page 113

hamstring
page 115

the cat
page 78

prayer
page 79

pilates for jet lag

Traveling to a different time zone is always a difficult adjustment to make, and this is usually compounded by aching shoulders from carrying heavy luggage and stiffness from sitting in a cramped airplane seat for many hours. Taking a little time for Pilates stretching will help overcome these discomforts, rebalancing the body, releasing tension, enhancing the breathing, and improving the circulation.

Other things you can do to help jet lag are:
• Avoid caffeine and alcohol—both are diuretics that will compound the dehydration you suffer from an airplane's air conditioning.
• Try not to graze. On long flights, meals and snacks are regularly provided, but they often have little nutritional content and can tempt you into eating out of boredom, leaving you feeling sluggish.
• Set your watch to the time zone you're traveling to. This will help you adjust to a new routine before you've arrived at your destination.

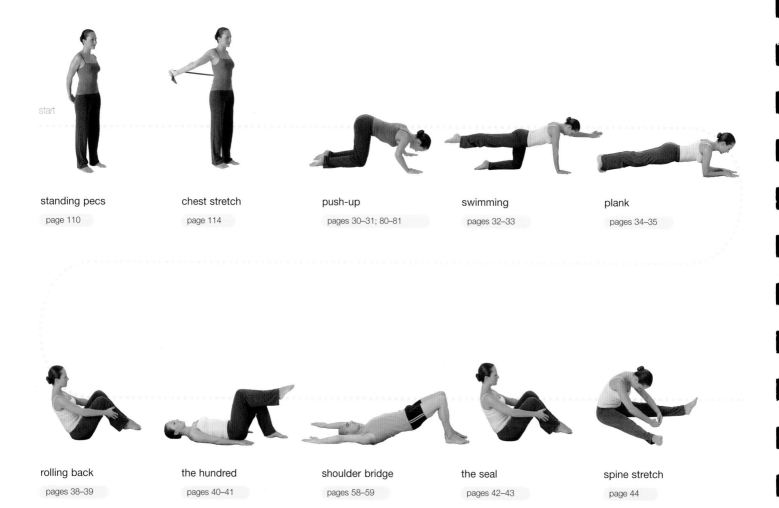

start

standing pecs

page 110

chest stretch

page 114

push-up

pages 30–31; 80–81

swimming

pages 32–33

plank

pages 34–35

rolling back

pages 38–39

the hundred

pages 40–41

shoulder bridge

pages 58–59

the seal

pages 42–43

spine stretch

page 44

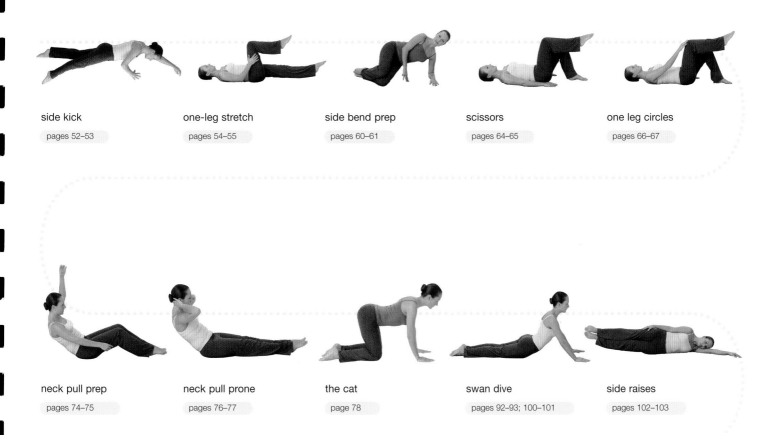

side kick

pages 52–53

one-leg stretch

pages 54–55

side bend prep

pages 60–61

scissors

pages 64–65

one leg circles

pages 66–67

neck pull prep

pages 74–75

neck pull prone

pages 76–77

the cat

page 78

swan dive

pages 92–93; 100–101

side raises

pages 102–103

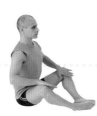

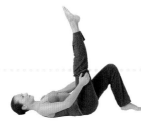

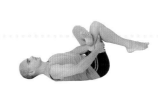

finish

inner thigh stretch

page 109

hamstring stretch

page 115

glute stretch

page 108

pilates for women

The Pilates system can be adapted to improve your general health, fitness, and vitality, whatever stage of life you are experiencing. Whether you have just reached adolescence, are planning on starting a family, recovering from childbirth, undergoing menopause, or enjoying old age, Pilates will help keep your body fit, healthy, and strong, improving your feeling of well-being and raising your self-esteem. If you are currently pregnant, seek medical advice before starting any program of exercise. It is probably best to wait until after the birth of your baby. Avoid exercising if you are between eight to sixteen weeks pregnant, as this is when you are at the highest risk of miscarriage. Check with your medical advisor before continuing with your exercises once again.

below left: Regular exercise for women of any age can help guard against osteoporosis.

below right: Exercising with a friend can help make your fitness routine much more fun.

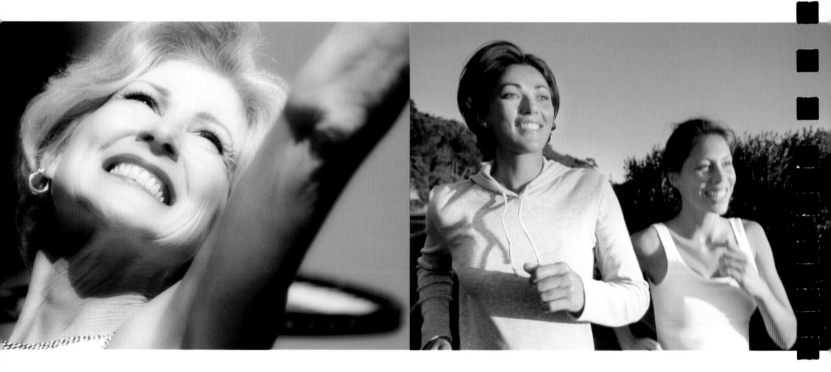

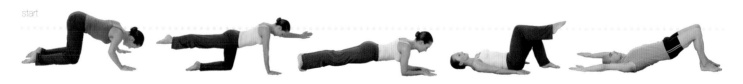

start

| push-up | swimming | plank | the hundred | shoulder bridge |
| pages 30–31; 80–81 | pages 32–33 | pages 34–35 | pages 40–41 | pages 58–59 |

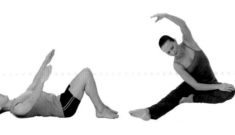

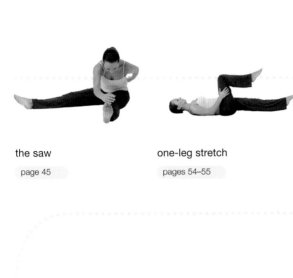

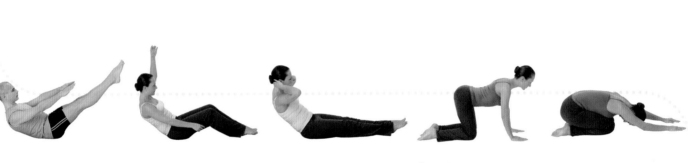

the saw

page 45

one-leg stretch

pages 54–55

double arm stretch 1

pages 56–57

side bend stretch

page 63

one leg circles

pages 66–67

teaser

pages 72–73

neck pull prep

pages 74–75

neck pull prone

pages 76–77

the cat

page 78

prayer

page 79

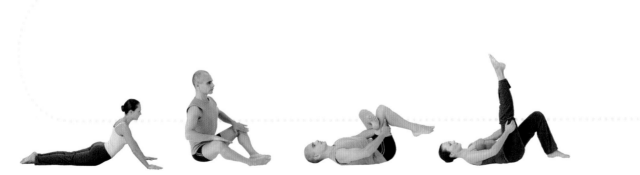

finish

swan dive

pages 92–93; 100–101

inner thigh stretch

page 109

glute stretch

page 108

hamstring

page 115

pilates for men

The benefits of the Pilates technique for men are considerable. Pilates offers a method of strength training that strengthens and stretches the body, while improving breathing, posture, and circulation. Although it is not a cardiovascular form of exercise, it is excellent for the heart and provides the perfect complement to other fitness programs. It also has the added benefit of reducing stress and relaxing the mind and body.

Some pointers for men starting a fitness program are:
• Don't forget to include cardiovascular exercise in your routine. Men are often tempted to concentrate on muscle growth, but it is essential to exercise your heart and lungs for true health and fitness.
• Always check in with a doctor before starting an exercise routine.
• Don't compete with other people. Listen to your own body and only push yourself as far as feels comfortable.

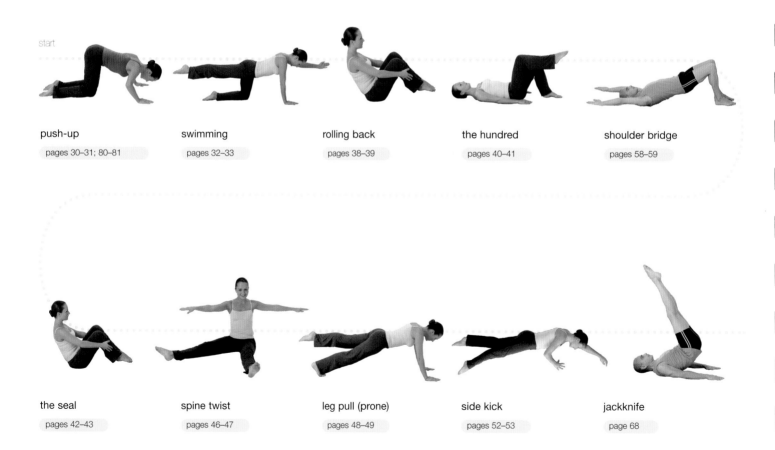

start

push-up
pages 30–31; 80–81

swimming
pages 32–33

rolling back
pages 38–39

the hundred
pages 40–41

shoulder bridge
pages 58–59

the seal
pages 42–43

spine twist
pages 46–47

leg pull (prone)
pages 48–49

side kick
pages 52–53

jackknife
page 68

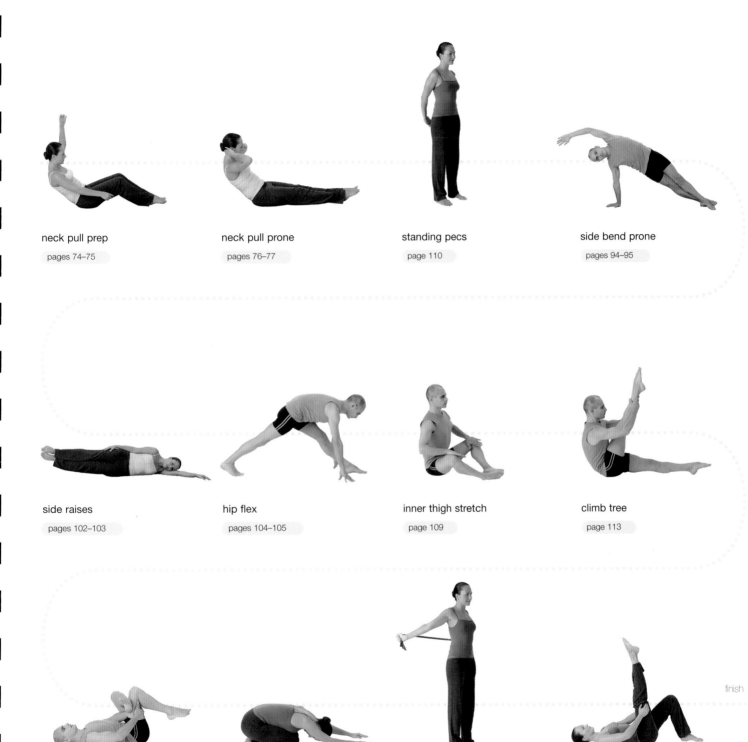

neck pull prep

pages 74–75

neck pull prone

pages 76–77

standing pecs

page 110

side bend prone

pages 94–95

side raises

pages 102–103

hip flex

pages 104–105

inner thigh stretch

page 109

climb tree

page 113

glute stretch

page 108

prayer

page 79

chest stretch

page 114

hamstring

page 115

finish

pilates for seniors

The beauty of Pilates is that it is suitable for everyone, regardless of age or level of fitness. Seniors who include a few minutes of Pilates stretching into their daily routine will benefit enormously—Pilates will encourage them to stay strong, supple, and trim. It will also enhance their general health, improving breathing and circulation and boosting the immune system. Developing a strong, healthy body will also mean that the internal organs are able to function more effectively. It is never too late to start exercising, and even for those who have recently come to realize the importance of a level of fitness, the gentle stretches of the Pilates technique are the perfect place to start.

Weight-bearing exercise has also been proven to help prevent osteoporosis and may be useful in the treatment of this condition. Several of the Pilates exercises can be done with light weights. If you do suffer from osteoporosis, however, consult your medical advisor before embarking on any program of exercise, and consult an experienced Pilates instructor to help devise the most appropriate program for you.

below left: A good social life can bring mental and physical benefits to older adults.

below right: Healthy, low-fat eating is crucial as you get older.

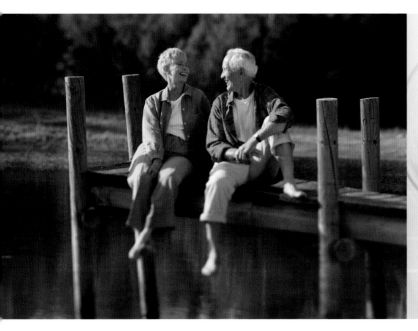
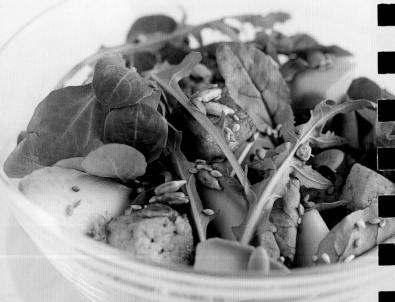

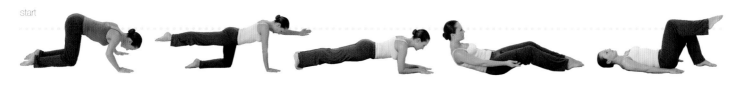

start

| push-up | swimming | plank | roll up | the hundred |
| pages 30–31 | pages 32–33 | pages 34–35 | pages 36–37 | pages 40–41 |

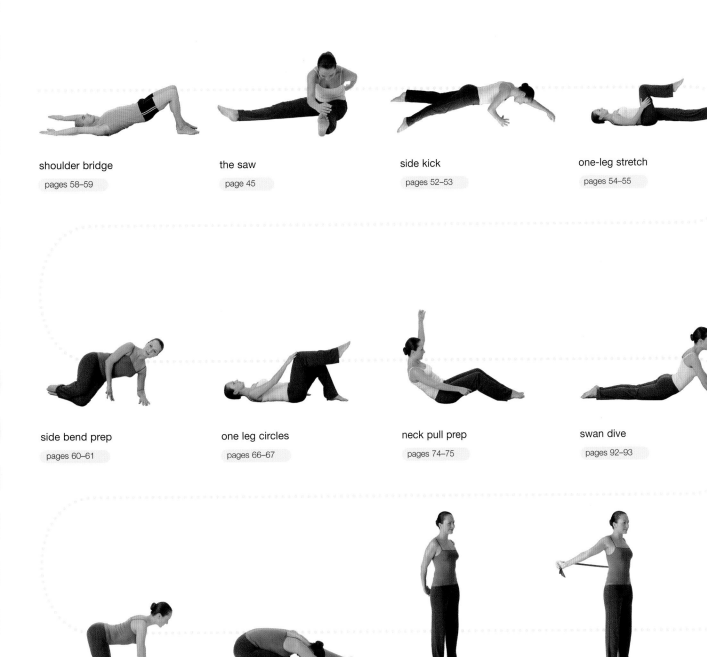

shoulder bridge

pages 58–59

the saw

page 45

side kick

pages 52–53

one-leg stretch

pages 54–55

side bend prep

pages 60–61

one leg circles

pages 66–67

neck pull prep

pages 74–75

swan dive

pages 92–93

the cat

page 78

prayer

page 79

standing pecs

page 110

chest stretch

page 114

finish

pilates for children

It is never too early to start looking after your body. Children can be just as prone to stresses and strains as adults, and learning good habits when we are young will greatly benefit us as we grow older. Children spend hours sitting behind desks and poring over books, carry heavy backpacks, and risk injuries playing sports. They suffer particular pressures at exam times, as well as having to cope with the pressures of growing up. Pilates offers children of all ages a method of rebalancing their bodies and gently stretching and strengthening their young muscles and joints. Improved fitness levels will also lead to better general health and greater resistance to colds.

below left: You're never too young to start doing regular exercise.

below right: Making food fun encourages children to eat healthily.

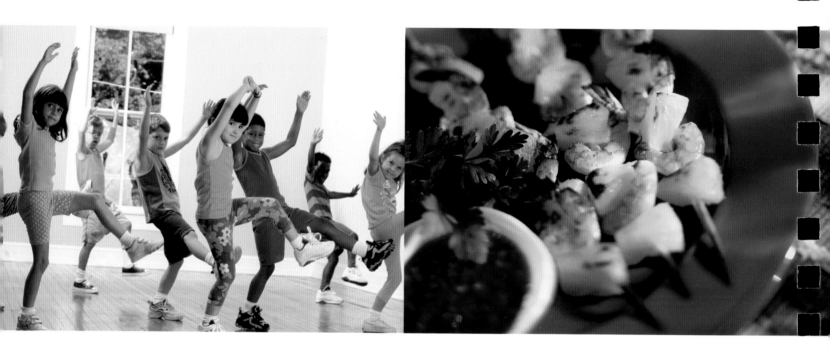

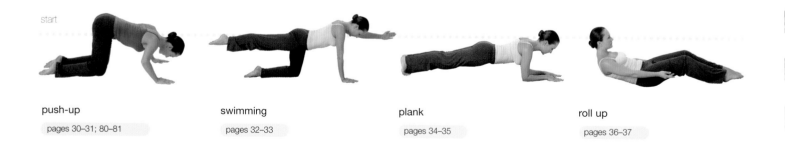

start

push-up

pages 30–31; 80–81

swimming

pages 32–33

plank

pages 34–35

roll up

pages 36–37

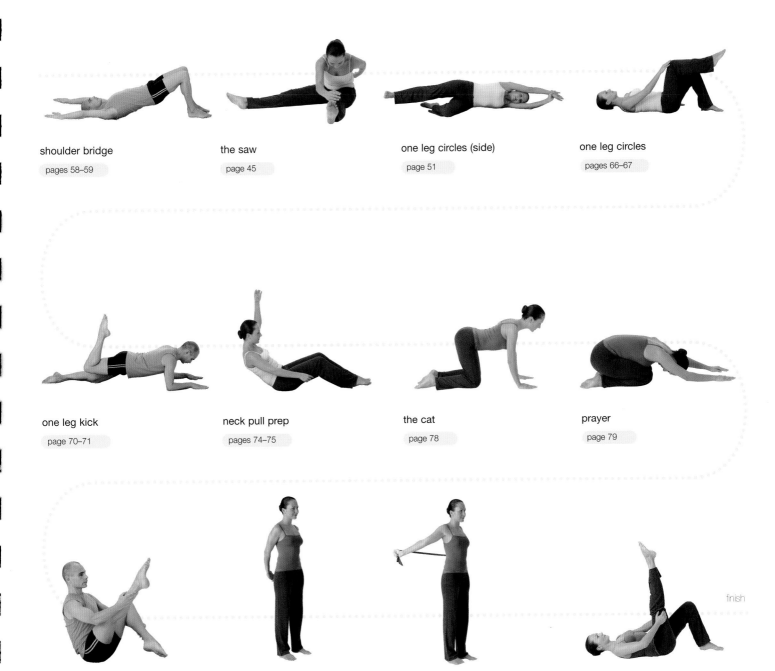

shoulder bridge

pages 58–59

the saw

page 45

one leg circles (side)

page 51

one leg circles

pages 66–67

one leg kick

page 70–71

neck pull prep

pages 74–75

the cat

page 78

prayer

page 79

open leg rocker

pages 82–83

standing pecs

page 110

chest stretch

page 114

hamstring

page 115

finish

taking it further

The series of Pilates mat-work moves offers you an extremely thorough program of exercises, which you can do in the privacy of your own home, organizing your exercise sessions to fit around your personal schedule. You can choose a short daily session (fifteen to twenty minutes), a slightly longer session two or three times a week (thirty to forty minutes), or one longer weekly session (sixty to ninety minutes).

With the growing interest in the Pilates system, there is an ever-increasing number of excellent books, videos, and DVDs available on the market today (see pages 187–189), focusing on different methods and aspects of Pilates. There are even books giving a combination of Pilates and other exercise systems such as bodybuilding and yoga. These will expand your knowledge and understanding of Pilates still further, and give you options for developing the method to suit your own particular requirements and preferences.

Remember: If you are recovering from illness or injury, are pregnant, or have recently lost or gained weight, you must seek medical advice before undertaking any exercise program. You should also consider attending classes under the guidance of a qualified Pilates instructor—making sure you inform them of any special needs or complaints you have.

If you enjoy practicing the Pilates technique, but are not content with exercising on your own or want to expand your knowledge, there are many excellent classes and courses now available to you. Although you can successfully work out at home, learning with a teacher to guide you is, for most people, infinitely more beneficial. So even if you plan to continue working out alone, you might consider undertaking at least a short course of Pilates classes.

Today, Pilates classes are widely available. There are many Pilates studios and most fitness centers offer classes. Most instructors offer the option of either group or private sessions.

Under Joseph Pilates' original system, half his session-time was devoted to mat-work, and the other half to moves carried out with the aid of his specially designed exercise equipment. The Pilates method is completely effective when carried out as a system of purely mat-work moves, but for those who prefer, there is the option of attending a Pilates studio and working with the special equipment under the guidance of an experienced instructor. The disadvantage of this system is that studio sessions tend to be much more expensive than mat-work classes.

Remember, whatever system you choose, it is only with your ongoing commitment to a regular routine of exercise, healthy eating, and sufficient rest that you can bring about permanent, positive changes to your body shape, level of fitness, and general well-being.

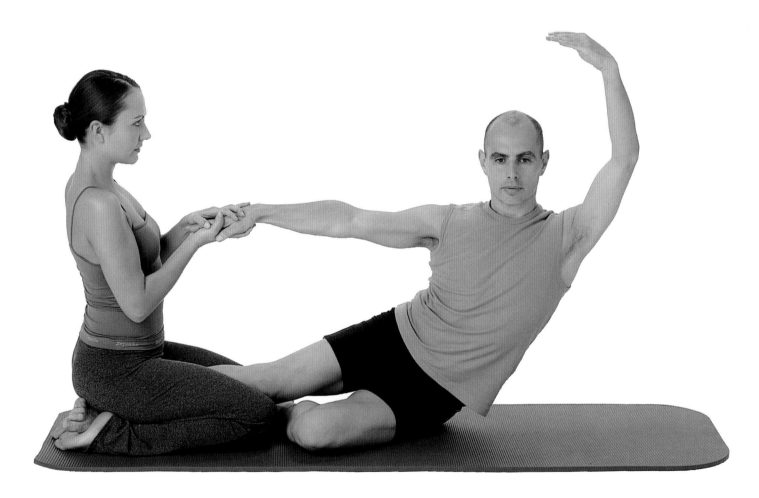

above: Working with a partner or the guidance of a teacher can help you develop your Pilates experience.

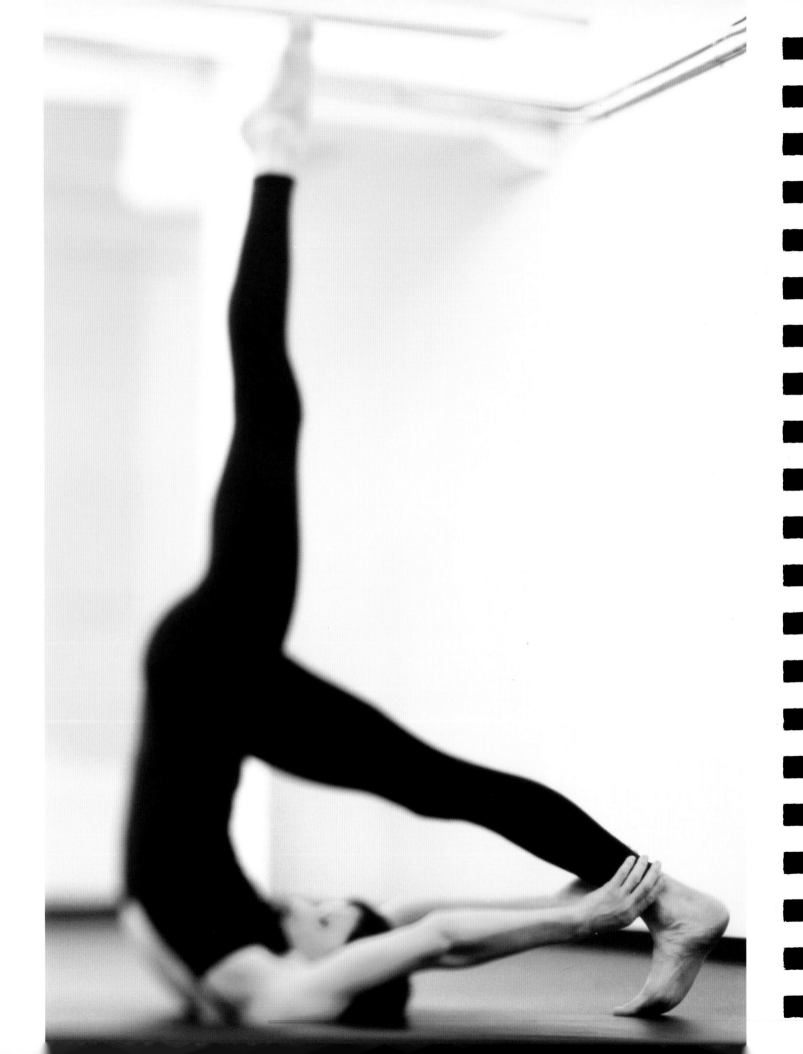

useful information

further reading

- Abdominal Training, *Christopher M. Norris*
- Body Control: The Pilates Way, *Lynne Robinson*
- Bounce Back Into Shape After Baby, *Caroline Corning Creager*
- Every Body Is Beautiful, *Ron Fletcher*
- How to Improve Your Posture, *Fran Lehen*
- Intelligent Exercise with Pilates & Yoga, *Lynne Robinson and Howard Napper*
- The Pilates Body, *Brooke Siler*
- Pilates for Beginners, *Roger Brignell*
- Pilates for Pregnancy, *Anna Selby*
- Pilates for Pregnancy, *Michael King and Yolande Green*
- Pilates Gym, *Lynne Robinson and Gerry Convy*
- Pilates on the Ball: The World's Most Popular Workout Using the Exercise Ball, *Colleen Craig*
- Pilates Powerhouse, *Mari Winsor and Mark Laska*
- The Pilates Pregnancy, *Mari Winsor and Mark Laska*
- Pure Pilates, *Michael King*
- The Body Control Pilates Back Book, *Lynne Robinson*
- The Official Body Control Fitness Manual, *Lynne Robinson*
- Therapeutic Exercises Using Foam Rollers, *Caroline Corning Creager*
- Therapeutic Exercises Using Resistive Bands, *Caroline Corning Creager*
- Therapeutic Exercises Using the Swiss Ball, *Caroline Corning Creager*

CD books

The following CD books are available from The Pilates Institute, and can be purchased online at www.pilates-institute.co.uk

- Pilates for Life—Pilates for Overall Fitness
- Pilates for Life—Pilates for Better Posture
- Pilates for Life—Pilates for Stress and Relaxation
- Pilates for Life—Pilates for Abdominal Strength
- Pilates for Life—Pilates for Sacroiliac Joints
- Pilates for Life—Pilates for Hips and Knees
- Pilates for Life—Pilates for Stronger Low Back
- Pilates for Life—Pilates for Neck and Shoulders
- Pilates for Life—Pilates for Firmer Bottoms
- Pilates for Life—Pilates for Pregnancy
- Pilates for Life—Pilates for Post Natal Strength
- Pilates for Life—Pilates for 50 Plus
- Pilates for Life—Pilates for Seniors
- Pilates for Life—Pilates for Scoliosis
- Pilates for Life—Pilates for Repetitive Strain Injury
- Pilates for Life—Pilates for Osteoporosis
- Pilates for Life—Pilates for Osteoarthritis
- Pilates for Life—Pilates for Golf
- Pilates for Life—Pilates for Racquet Sports
- Pilates for Life—Pilates for Driving

useful addresses

U.S.A

AB Studio
33 Bleecker Street
Suite 2C
New York
NY 10012
tel: (+1) 212 420 9111
website: www.reabnyc.com

Tribeca Bodyworks
177 Duane Street
New York
NY 10013
tel: (+1) 212 625 0777
fax: (+1) 212 625 0030
website: www.tribecabodyworks.com

Ultimate Body Control
30 East Sixtieth Street #606
New York
NY 10022
website: www.pilates-ny.com

Pilates Plus
409 Grand Avenue
Suite 2
Englewood
NJ 07631
tel: (+1) 201 569 7970
website: www.pilatesplus.org

Pilates Studio of Los Angeles
8704 Santa Monica Boulevard
Suite 300
West Hollywood
CA 90069
tel: (+1) 310 659 1077
website: www.pilatestherapy.com

U.K.

The Pilates Institute
3rd Floor
Wimborne House
151–155 New North Road
London N1 6TA
Tel: (+44) (0) 20 7253 3177
fax: (+44) (0) 20 7253 3144
e-mail: info@pilates-institute.co.uk
website: www.pilates-institute.co.uk

The Body Control Pilates Association
P.O. Box 29061
London WC2H 9TB
website: www.bodycontrol.co.uk

The Pilates Foundation U.K. Ltd.
P.O. Box 36052
London SW16 1XQ
tel: (+44) (0) 7071 781559
fax: (+44) (0) 20 8696 0088
e-mail: admin@pilatesfoundation.com
website: www.pilatesfoundation.com

The Alan Herdman Studio
17 Homer Row
London W1H 4AP
tel: (+44) (0) 20 7723 9953

Body Maintenance Studio
2nd Floor
Pineapple Studios
7 Langley Street
London WC2H 9JA

music CDs

The following CDs can be purchased online from New World Music at www.newworldmusic.com

Celestial Guardian, Philip Chapman (New World Music)
Crystal Healing, Anthony Miles (New World Music)
Music for Relaxation, Philip Chapman, Anthony Miles, and Stephen Rhodes (New World Music)
Pilates, Llewellyn (New World Music)
Temple of Healing, Anthony Miles (New World Music)

exercise videos/DVDs

- Introduction to Pilates—The Power Within
- Isotoner Workout Volume 1, Michael King, Pilates Institute
- Pilates Express, Lynne Robinson and Pat Cash
- Pilates Intermediate Matwork—Volume 1, Pilates Institute
- Pilates Matwork Volume 1 Pilates Institute
- Pilates Matwork Volume 2, Pilates Institute
- Pilates Matwork, Progressions, Pilates Institute
- Pilates on the Ball, Pilates Institute
- Pilates Powerhouse, Body Control 5 with Lynne Robinson
- Pilates, Micah Bo, Int.
- Pilates: The Perfect Body & Pilates Express
- Pilates-Inspired Matwork—Volumes 1–3
- Roll Up to Unwind—Fitball Flexibility & Mobility, Lisa Westlake, Pilates Institute
- Super Sculpt, Michael King, Pilates Institute
- Tripower, Michael King, Pilates Institute
- Yogalates

websites

www.allaboutpilates.com
www.backpain.org
www.balancedbody.com
www.bodymind.net
www.bodyzone.com
www.classicalpilates.net
www.excelpilates.com
www.gothampilates.com
www.jumpingtiger.com
www.newworldmusic.com
www.physicalcompany.co.uk
www.physioworks.co.uk
www.pilates.com
www.pilates.net
www.pilatesbodyworksintl.com
www.pilatesdirect.com
www.pilates-marybowen.com
www.pilatesontheball.com
www.pilates-studio.com
www.powerpilates.com
www.sagefitness.com
www.sissel-online.com
www.stottpilates.com
www.themethodpilates.com
www.thepilatescenter.com
www.thethirdspace.com
www.turningpointstudios.com
www.winsorpilates.com

index